HANDBOOK OF
DIABETES

HANDBOOK OF
DIABETES

EDITED BY

GARETH WILLIAMS MA, MD, FRCP

DEPARTMENT OF MEDICINE
LIVERPOOL UNIVERSITY
ROYAL LIVERPOOL HOSPITAL, LIVERPOOL
AND

JOHN C. PICKUP MA, DPhil, BM, BCh, MRCPath

DIVISION OF CHEMICAL PATHOLOGY
UNITED MEDICAL AND DENTAL SCHOOLS OF
GUY'S AND ST THOMAS'S HOSPITALS
GUY'S HOSPITAL, LONDON

OXFORD

BLACKWELL SCIENTIFIC PUBLICATIONS

LONDON EDINBURGH BOSTON

MELBOURNE PARIS BERLIN VIENNA

To Caroline, Timothy and Kim;
Selma, Matthew, Charlotte and Joshua

© 1992 by
Blackwell Scientific Publications
Editorial Offices:
Osney Mead, Oxford OX2 oEL
25 John Street, London WC1N 2BL
23 Ainslie Place, Edinburgh EH3 6AJ
3 Cambridge Center, Cambridge
    Massachusetts 02142, USA
54 University Street, Carlton
    Victoria 3053, Australia

Other Editorial Offices:
Arnette SA
2, rue Casimir-Delavigne
75006 Paris
France

Blackwell Wissenschaft
Meinekestrasse 4
D-1000 Berlin 15
Germany

Blackwell MZV
Feldgasse 13
A-1238 Wien
Austria

First published 1992

Set by Setrite Typesetters, Hong Kong
Printed and bound in Great Britain
by Cambridge University Press, Cambridge

DISTRIBUTORS

Marston Book Services Ltd
PO Box 87
Oxford OX2 oDT
(*Orders*: Tel: 0865 791155
        Fax: 0865 791927
        Telex: 837515)

USA
Mosby-Year Book, Inc.
11830 Westline Industrial Drive
St Louis, Missouri 63146
(*Orders*: Tel: 800 633–6699)

Canada
Mosby-Year Book, Inc.
5240 Finch Avenue East
Scarborough, Ontario
(*Orders*: Tel: 416 298–1588)

Australia
Blackwell Scientific Publications
(Australia) Pty Ltd
54 University Street
Carlton, Victoria 3053
(*Orders*: Tel: 03 347–0300)

British Library
Cataloguing in Publication Data

Handbook of diabetes.
  1. Humans. Diabetes
  I. Williams, Gareth 1952–
  II. Pickup, John C. (Christopher)
616.462

ISBN 0–632–02888–2

Contents

List of contributors
to the Textbook of Diabetes

A. MICHAEL ALBISSER, BEng, MA, PhD, *Loyal True Blue and Orange Research Institute, Ontario, Canada*

CLIFFORD J. BAILEY, BSc, PhD, *Aston University, Birmingham, UK*

PETER J. BARRY, FRCS, FCOphth, *Royal Victoria Eye and Ear Hospital and St Vincent's Hospital, Dublin, Ireland*

PETER H. BENNETT, MB, FRCP, FFCM, *National Institute of Diabetes and Digestive and Kidney Diseases, Phoenix, USA*

D. JOHN BETTERIDGE, BSc, MD, PhD, FRCP, *University College and Middlesex School of Medicine, London, UK*

RUDOLF W. BILOUS, MD, MRCP, *The Medical School, Newcastle upon Tyne, UK*

CHRISTIAN BINDER, MD, *Steno Memorial and Hvidøre Hospital, Gentofte, Denmark*

ANNE E. BISHOP, PhD, *Royal Postgraduate Medical School, London, UK*

MICHAEL BLISS, MA, PhD, FRSC, *University of Toronto, Toronto, Canada*

STEPHEN R. BLOOM, DSc, MD, FRCP, *Royal Postgraduate Medical School, London, UK*

GEREMIA B. BOLLI, MD, *Istituto Patologica Medica, Perugia, Italy*

ADRIAN J. BONE, BSc, DPhil, *Southampton General Hospital, Southampton, UK*

EZIO BONIFACIO, BSc, PhD, *University College and Middlesex School of Medicine, London, UK*

KNUT BORSH-JOHNSEN, MD, *Steno Memorial Hospital, Gentofte, Denmark*

GIAN FRANCO BOTTAZZO, MD, FRCP, *University College and Middlesex School of Medicine, London, UK*

MICHAEL BROWNLEE, MD, *Albert Einstein College of Medicine, The Bronx, New York, USA*

RAYMOND BRUCE, MB, ChB, *Wynn Institute for Metabolic Research, London, UK*

TERENCE CHADWICK, BSc, MB, ChB, MRCP, MFPP, *Fisons PLC, Loughborough, Leicestershire, UK*

AH WAH CHAN, MB, BCh, MRCP (UK), *Royal Liverpool Hospital, Liverpool, UK*

CHI KONG CHING, MB, ChB, MRCP, *Senior Derbyshire Royal Infirmary, Derby, UK*

DONALD J. CHISHOLM, MB, BS, FRACP, *St Vincent's Hospital, Sydney, Australia*

PENELOPE M. S. CLARK, PhD, MRCPath, *Addenbrooke's Hospital, Cambridge, UK*

BASIL F. CLARKE, MB, FRCPE, *The Royal Infirmary, Edinburgh, UK*

PHILIP COHEN, BSc, PhD, *University of Dundee, Dundee, UK*

CAROLINE J. CRACE, PhD, *Northern General Hospital, Sheffield, UK*

ADRIAN J. CRISP, MA, MD, MRCP (UK), *Addenbrooke's Hospital, Cambridge, UK*

JOHN L. DAY, MD, FRCP, *The Ipswich Hospital, Ipswich, UK*

TORSTEN DECKERT, MD, DMSc, *Steno Memorial Hospital, Gentofte, Denmark*

JOHN DUPRÉ, FRCP (Lond.), FRCP (C), *University Hospital London, Ontario, Canada*

MICHAEL E. EDMONDS, MD, MRCP, *King's College Hospital, London, UK*

JEAN-MARIE EKOÉ, MD, *University of Montréal, Montréal, Canada*

DAVID J. EWING, MD, FRCP, *The Royal Infirmary, Edinburgh, UK*

PETER R. FLATT, BSc, PhD, *University of Ulster, Coleraine, Northern Ireland, UK*

ALI V. M. FOSTER, BA (Hons), DPodM, SRCh, *King's College Hospital, London, UK*

ALAN K. FOULIS, BSc, MD, MRCPath, *Royal Infirmary, Glasgow, UK*

BRIAN M. FRIER, BSc, MD, FRCP, *The Royal Infirmary, Edinburgh, UK*

GEOFFREY V. GILL, MSc, MD, FRCP, DTM & H, *Arrowe Park Hospital, Merseyside, UK*

BARRY J. GOLDSTEIN, MD, PhD, *Harvard Medical School, Boston, USA*

DEREK W. R. GRAY, DPhil, FRCS, MRCP, *John Radcliffe Hospital, Oxford, UK*

STEPHEN A. GREENE, MB, BS, MRCP, *Ninewells Hospital and Medical School, Dundee, UK*

ANASUYA GRENFELL, MA, MD, MRCP, *Ipswich Hospital, Ipswich, UK*

C. NICK HALES, MA, MD, PhD, FRCPath FRCP, *Addenbrooke's Hospital, Cambridge, UK*

KRISTIAN F. HANSSEN, MD, *Aker Hospital, Oslo, Norway*

D. GRAHAME HARDIE, MA, PhD, *University of Dundee, Dundee, UK*

SUSAN E. HILL, *Toronto General Hospital, Toronto, Canada*

GRAHAM A. HITMAN, MB, FRCP, *The Royal London Hospital, London, UK*

RURY R. HOLMAN, MB, ChB, MRCP (UK), *Radcliffe Infirmary, Oxford, UK*

PHILIP D. HOME, MA, DPhil, FRCP, *Freeman Hospital, Newcastle upon Tyne, UK*

SIMON L. HOWELL, BSc, PhD, DSc, *King's College, London, UK*

STEPHEN L. HYER, MD, MRCP, *St George's Hospital, London, UK*

KARL IRSIGLER, MD, *City Hospital Vienna-Lainz, Vienna, Austria*

JAMES G. L. JACKSON, MD, (h.c.) *European Association for the Study of Diabetes, Chertsey, Surrey, UK*

R. JOHN JARRETT, MD, FFCM, *United Medical and Dental Schools, Guy's Campus, London, UK*

ROGER H. JAY, MA, MB, BS, MRCP, *University College and Middlesex School of Medicine, London, UK*

PATRICIA M. JOHNS, RN, RM, *Dip. Nursing, Maidstone Hospital, Maidstone, UK*

DESMOND G. JOHNSTON, FRCP, PhD, *St. Mary's Hospital Medical School, London, UK*

JACQUELINE N. JONES, BSc, SRN, *Greenwich District Hospital, London, UK*

RICHARD H. JONES, MA, MB, FRCP, *Senior Lecturer, Medway Hospital, Gillingham, UK*

C. RONALD KAHN, MD, *Harvard Medical School, Boston, USA*

HARRY KEEN, MD, FRCP, *United Medical and Dental Schools, Guy's Campus, London, UK*

LAURENCE KENNEDY, MD, FRCP, *Royal Victoria Hospital, Belfast, Northern Ireland, UK*

RONALD KLEIN, MD, MPH, *University of Wisconsin, Madison, USA*

ANTHONY H. KNIGHT, FRCP, *Stoke Mandeville Hospital, Aylesbury, UK*

EVA M. KOHNER, MD, FRCP, *Royal Postgraduate Medical School, London, UK*

VEIKKO A. KOIVISTO, MD, *Helsinki University Second Hospital, Helsinki, Finland*

EDWARD W. KRAEGEN, BSc, PhD, *St Vincents Hospital, Sydney, Australia*

BERNHARD KREYMANN, MD, *ii. Medizinische Klinik und Poliklinik Der Technischen Universität München, München, Germany*

A. J. KRENTZ, MB, ChB, MRCP, *The General Hospital, Birmingham, UK*

ANTONY KURTZ, PhD, FRCP, *University College and Middlesex School of Medicine, London, UK*

MIKE E. J. LEAN, MA, MD, FRCP, *Royal Infirmary, Glasgow, UK*

DAVID LESLIE, MD, FRCP, *Charing Cross and Westminster Medical School, London, UK*

BIRGITTA LINDE, MD, PhD, *Karolinska Hospital, Stockholm, Sweden*

WILLIAM D. LOUGHEED, PEng, *Loyal True Blue and Orange Research Institute, Ontario, Canada*

CLARA LOWY, MB, MSc, FRCP, *St Thomas's Hospital, London, UK*

DAVID R. MCCANCE, BSc, MD, MRCP, *Royal Victoria Hospital, Belfast, Northern Ireland, UK*

IAN A. MACFARLANE, MD, MRCP, *Walton Hospital, Liverpool, UK*

TERESA MCLEAN, MA (Oxon), *Cricket Journalist, 31 Newmarket Road, Cambridge, UK*

ANDREW MACLEOD, MA, MRCP, *St Thomas's Hospital, London, UK*

ALASDAIR MCLEOD, BSc, BDS, *Birkbeck College, London, UK*

J. L. MAHON, MD, FRCP (C), *University Hospital London, Ontario, Canada*

JIM I. MANN, MA, DM, PhD, *University of Otago, Dunedin, New Zealand*

BRENDAN MARSHALL, PhD, *The London Hospital, London, UK*

HUGH M. MATHER, MD, FRCP, *Ealing Hospital, Southall, Middlesex, UK*

V. MOHAN, MD, MNAMS, PhD, *Diabetes Research Centre, Royapuram, Madras, India*

PETER J. MORRIS, PhD, FRCS, FRACS, FACS (Hon.), *John Radcliffe Hospital, Oxford, UK*

CATHLEEN J. MULLARKEY, MD, *Albert Einstein College of Medicine, The Bronx, New York, USA*

MALCOLM NATTRASS, MB, ChB, PhD, FRCP, *The General Hospital, Birmingham, UK*

JOHN C. PICKUP, MA, BM, DPhil, MRCPath, *Division of Chemical Pathology, United Medical and Dental Schools of Guy's and St Thomas's Hospitals, Guy's Hospital, London SE1 9RT, UK*

JULIA M. POLAK, DSc, MD, FRCPath, *Royal Postgraduate Medical School, London, UK*

MASSIMO PORTA, MD, PhD, *University of Sassari, Italy*

A. RAMACHANDRAN, MD, MNAMS, PhD, *Diabetes Research Centre, Royapuram, Madras, India*

LUIS C. RAMIREZ, MD, *University of Texas Southwestern Medical Center, Dallas, USA*

PHILIP RASKIN, MD, *University of Texas Southwestern Medical Center, Dallas, USA*

S. SETHU K. REDDY, MD, FRCPC, *Dalhousie University, Halifax, Canada*

JONATHAN M. RHODES, MA, MD, FRCP, *Royal Liverpool Hospital, Liverpool, UK*

PATRICK SHARP, MD, MRCP, *St. Mary's Hospital Medical School, London, UK*

GARY R. SIBBALD, BSc, MD, FRCP (C), ABIM, DAAD, *Women's College Hospital, University of Toronto, Toronto, Canada*

ANGELA C. SHORE, BSc, PhD, *Royal Devon & Exeter Hospital, Exeter, UK*

JUDITH M. STEEL, MB ChB, FRCPEd, *Edinburgh Royal Infirmary, Edinburgh, UK*

JOHN C. STEVENSON, MB, MRCP, *Wynn Institute for Metabolic Research, London, UK*

C. R. STILLER, MD, FRCP (C), *University of Western Ontario; Ontario, Canada*

ROBERT W. STOUT, MD, DSc, FRCP, FRCPEd, FRCPI, *The Queen's University of Belfast, Belfast, Northern Ireland, UK*

ROBERT SUTTON, MB, BS, FRCS, DPhil (Oxon), *John Radcliffe Hospital, Oxford, UK*

TERESA M. SZOPA, BSc, PhD, *London Hospital, London, UK*

HOWARD S. TAGER, PhD, *The University of Chicago, Chicago, USA*

PETER R. W. TASKER, MB, BS, DCH, FRCGP, *Doomsday House, South Wootton, Norfolk, UK*

ROBERT B. TATTERSALL, MD, FRCP, *University Hospital, Nottingham, UK*

KEITH W. TAYLOR, MA, PhD, MRCP, *London Hospital, Whitechapel, London, UK*

ROY TAYLOR, BSc, MD, FRCP, *Royal Victoria Infirmary, Newcastle upon Tyne, UK*

P. K. THOMAS, DSc, MD, FRCP, FRCPath, *Royal Free Hospital School of Medicine, London, UK*

JOHN E. TOOKE, MA, MSc, DM, MRCP, *Royal Devon and Exeter Hospital, Exeter, UK*

ROBERT C. TURNER, MD, FRCP, *Radcliffe Infirmary, Oxford, UK*

GIAN CARLO VIBERTI, MD, FRCP, *United Medical and Dental Schools, Guy's Hospital Campus, London, UK*

M. VISWANATHAN, MD, FAMS, *Diabetes Research Centre, Royapuram, Madras, India*

JAMES D. WALKER, BSc, MRCP, *St Bartholomew's Hospital, London, UK*

JOHN D. WARD, BSc, MD, FRCP, *Royal Hallamshire Hospital, Sheffield, UK*

PER WESTERMARK, MD, *University of Uppsala, Uppsala, Sweden*

GREG WILKINSON, FRCP (Edin.), MRCPsych, *University of Wales College of Medicine, Denbigh, UK*

D.R.R. WILLIAMS, MA, PhD, MFPHM, *Addenbrooke's Hospital, Cambridge, UK*

GARETH WILLIAMS, MA, MD, FRCP, *Royal Liverpool Hospital, Liverpool, UK*

R. MALCOLM WILSON, DM, MRCP, *Royal Hallamshire Hospital, Sheffield, UK*

PETER H. WISE, MB, BS, PhD, FRCP, FRACP, *Charing Cross Hospital, London, UK*

STEVEN P. WOOD, BSc, DPhil, *Birkbeck College, London, UK*

Preface

The aim of this book is to summarize some of the information contained in its parent volume, the *Textbook of Diabetes*, which is also published by Blackwell Scientific Publications. Most of this Handbook is devoted to the day-to-day treatment and surveillance of diabetes and its commoner problems, and is biased deliberately towards health professionals with an interest in diabetes who work outside hospital. We have included sections on screening for diabetic complications (particularly retinopathy), on the treatment of lipid disorders and hypertension, and on topics such as contraception, driving, insurance and assistance for the partially sighted. There are also detailed accounts of the composition of the integrated diabetes care team and the roles of its various members, particularly the diabetes specialist nurse, and of ways of sharing the burden of diabetes care between hospital and the community. For these reasons, we hope that this book would be useful to those setting up or running a diabetic 'miniclinic' in a general practice setting.

At the same time, we recognize that our selection of topics has been personal, and perhaps even idiosyncratic. We have included several sections on the management of problems (such as surgery, coma and end-stage renal failure) which obviously remain in the province of the hospital specialist. We also make no apologies for including some detailed scientific topics such as the causes of diabetes and the metabolic basis of its complications. We have done this deliberately, to try to keep the reader aware of the immense medical, scientific and social impact of the disease and of the need to unite many different disciplines in the battle against its many problems.

Producing this Handbook has been, for us, a relatively painless exercise, mostly because of the excellence of the contributions to the parent Textbook from which the present material is distilled. We would therefore like to record our gratitude to the 120 authors of the original chapters in the Textbook; their names are listed on pages vi–viii and luckily, many of them have remained (or even become) our friends. We are also indebted to the team at Blackwell Scientific Publications — notably Julian Grover, Peter Saugman and Andrew Robinson — for their infectious enthusiasm and good humour, and to David Ray, for remaining outwardly cheerful while grappling with the proofs. Finally, it would be churlish and possibly risky for us not to thank our wives and families, who have supported us selflessly and generally exceeded the call of duty during the last three and a half years of editorial house arrest.

GARETH WILLIAMS
JOHN C. PICKUP
Liverpool and London, May 1991

1: Diagnosis and classification of diabetes mellitus

- The *diabetic syndrome* is characterized by chronic hyperglycaemia. Clinical features include symptoms and signs primarily related to the severity of the metabolic disturbance.
- The syndrome has several well-defined causes but those of the more common types are only partially understood.
- *The WHO classification* (1980 and 1985), based on the US National Diabetes Data Group recommendations, is now generally accepted (Table 1.1). Individuals fall within a single class (defined by simple clinical and biochemical descriptions) at any one time, but their classification may change in the course of time.
- *Insulin-dependent diabetes mellitus* (IDDM) and *non-insulin-dependent diabetes mellitus* (NIDDM) are distinguished by the propensity to develop ketosis and the dependency on insulin treatment for survival in the former class.
- *Malnutrition-related diabetes mellitus* occurs primarily in tropical developing countries and is associated with nutritional deficiency and the absence of spontaneous ketosis.
- *Other types of diabetes mellitus* are associated with well-defined conditions such as chronic pancreatitis, haemochromatosis, endocrine disorders, drug administration, mutant insulins and insulin receptor abnormalities (Table 1.2).
- *Gestational diabetes* is that which occurs for the first time during pregnancy.
- *Impaired glucose tolerance* (IGT) describes hyperglycaemia during an oral glucose tolerance test (OGTT), but below the levels diagnostic of diabetes. These subjects have an increased risk of developing diabetes subsequently and are vulnerable to macrovascular disease.
- *Statistical risk classes* describe currently normoglycaemic individuals who either have had a previous abnormality of glucose tolerance (e.g. gestational diabetes or IGT), or have a potential abnormality (e.g. normal subjects with islet cell antibodies, human leukocyte-associated antigen-identical siblings of diabetic patients). Both classes are at increased risk of developing diabetes.

Table 1.1. 1985 WHO (World Health Organization) classification of diabetes mellitus and allied categories of glucose intolerance.

A. CLINICAL CLASSES
Diabetes mellitus
- *Insulin-dependent diabetes mellitus (IDDM)*
- *Non-insulin-dependent diabetes mellitus (NIDDM)*
  (a) Non-obese
  (b) Obese
- *Malnutrition-related diabetes mellitus (MRDM)*
- *Other types of diabetes mellitus* associated with specific conditions and syndromes (see Table 1.2 for details)
- *Gestational diabetes mellitus (GDM)*

Impaired glucose tolerance (IGT)
(a) Non-obese
(b) Obese
(c) Associated with certain conditions and syndromes

B. STATISTICAL RISK CLASSES
Previous abnormality of glucose tolerance
Potential abnormality of glucose tolerance

Table 1.2. Other types of diabetes mellitus.

1 Diabetes due to pancreatic disease
  - Chronic or recurrent pancreatitis
  - Haemochromatosis

2 Diabetes due to other endocrine disease
  - Cushing's syndrome
  - Hyperaldosteronism
  - Acromegaly
  - Thyrotoxicosis
  - Phaeochromocytoma
  - Glucagonoma

3 Diabetes due to drugs and toxins
  - Glucocorticoids and ACTH
  - Diazoxide
  - Diuretics
  - Phenytoin
  - Pentamidine
  - Vacor (rodenticide)

4 Diabetes due to abnormalities of insulin or its receptor
  - Insulinopathies
  - Receptor defects
  - Circulating antireceptor antibodies

5 Diabetes associated with genetic syndromes
  - DIDMOAD syndrome
  - Myotonic dystrophy and other muscle disorders
  - Lipoatrophy
  - Type 1 glycogen storage disease
  - Cystic fibrosis

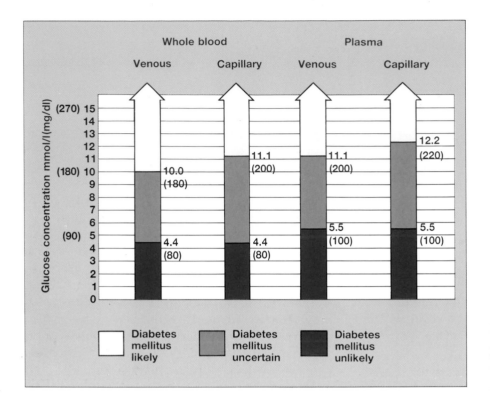

Fig. 1.1. Casual (random) blood glucose values and their interpretations. The corresponding values in mg/dl are shown in parentheses.

Table 1.3. Diagnostic values for diabetes using the oral glucose tolerance test.*

	Glucose concentration, mmol/l (mg/dl)			
	Whole blood		Plasma	
	Venous	Capillary	Venous	Capillary
Diabetes mellitus				
Fasting value	≥6.7	≥6.7	≥7.8	≥7.8
or	(≥120)	(≥120)	(≥140)	(≥140)
2 h after glucose load	≥10.0	≥11.1	11.1	≥12.2
	(≥180)	(≥200)	(≥200)	(≥220)
Impaired glucose tolerance				
Fasting value	<6.7	<6.7	<7.8	<7.8
and	(<120)	(<120)	(<140)	(<140)
2 h after glucose load	6.7−10.0	7.8−11.1	7.8−11.1	8.9−12.2
	(120−180)	(140−200)	(140−200)	(160−220)

* For epidemiological or population screening purposes the 2-h value after 75-g oral glucose may be used alone. The fasting value alone is considered less reliable since true fasting cannot be assured and the spurious diagnosis of diabetes may more readily occur.

● Diabetes can be diagnosed in *symptomatic patients* by a grossly elevated random blood, or plasma glucose concentration (Fig. 1.1), or by two fasting values above a specified range (whole blood glucose>6.7 mmol/l, or plasma glucose> 7.8 mmol/l).

● *When doubt exists,* a formal 75-g OGTT must be performed. The WHO diagnostic criteria applied to the venous plasma glucose level 2 h after the load define diabetes as >11.1 mmol/l, IGT as between 7.8 and 11.1 mmol/l, and normal glucose tolerance as <7.8 mmol/l (Table 1.3).

● *Urinary glucose,* or glycated haemoglobin (HbA$_1$) or other glycated protein measurements, *should not be used to diagnose diabetes.*

2: The clinical problem of insulin-dependent diabetes mellitus

- Insulin-dependent diabetes mellitus (IDDM), generally synonymous with Type 1 diabetes, identifies patients who cannot survive without insulin replacement.
- The prevalence of IDDM in the UK is about 0.25%; there is marked geographical variation in its prevalence world-wide.
- The incidence of IDDM peaks at about 11–13 years of age (Fig. 2.1).
- There is a striking seasonal variation in incidence in older children and adolescents, with lowest rates in the spring and summer (Fig. 2.2).
- Incidence varies enormously between countries, being 35 times higher in Finland than in Japan.
- The incidence is increasing in some countries (Finland and Scotland) but apparently not in others (USA).
- Patients mostly present young but over 10% of diabetic subjects aged over 65 years require insulin.
- IDDM usually presents acutely with hyperglycaemic symptoms (polyuria, thirst, polydipsia), tiredness and weight loss. Nausea, vomiting and drowsiness usually denote impending keto-acidosis. Minor symptoms include cramps, blurred vision and superficial infections (Table 2.1).
- The acute presentation of IDDM is probably the culmination of chronic autoimmune destruction of the pancreatic B-cells. Subtle abnormalities of insulin secretion and glucose tolerance can be detected during this 'prediabetic' phase.
- Some IDDM patients experience a temporary remission ('honeymoon period') after starting insulin, with good glycaemic control and low insulin requirements (Fig. 2.3). This is due to correction of hyperglycaemia, which directly damages the B-cells. Remission ends when continuing autoimmune damage has destroyed a critical mass of B-cells.
- Long-standing IDDM patients are susceptible to 'microvascular' complications (nephropathy, retinopathy and neuropathy) specific to diabetes

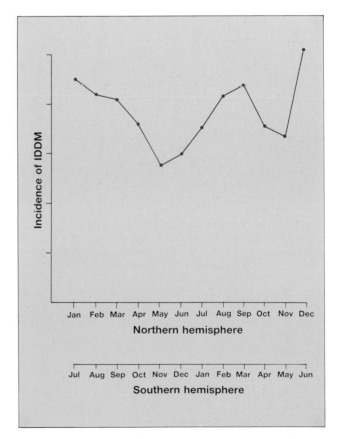

Fig. 2.2. Seasonal pattern of incidence of the clinical onset of IDDM in children and adolescents. One suggested explanation for this is the variation in the frequency of viral infections at different times of the year—a positive trigger for the development of IDDM.

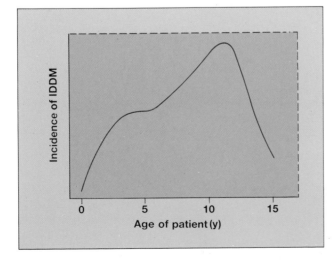

Fig. 2.1. Variation in IDDM incidence with age, showing the peak at 11–13 years.

Major symptoms	Minor symptoms	Features of ketoacidosis
Thirst	Cramps	Nausea
Polyuria	Constipation	Vomiting
Weight loss	Blurred vision	Drowsiness
Fatigue	Candidiasis	Abdominal pain
	Skin sepsis	

Table 2.1. Symptoms of insulin-dependent diabetes (IDDM). NB: Symptoms due to diabetic microvascular complications are extremely rare at presentation.

Duration of DM (y)	Neuropathy (%)	Retinopathy (%)	Nephropathy (%)
0	8	5	0
5	15	16	2
10	26	26	5
15	31	40	8
20	40	48	10
25	49	50	14

Table 2.2. Percentage of patients affected by different diabetic complications with increasing duration of diabetes.

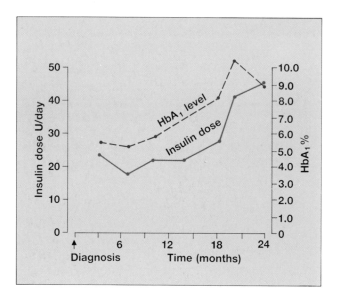

Fig. 2.3. The 'honeymoon period' in a teenager with IDDM. The graph shows daily insulin dose and glycosylated haemoglobin (HbA$_1$) levels in an 18-year-old girl during the first 2 years after diagnosis. Insulin requirements fell in the first 6 months, typical of the honeymoon period. Glycaemic control then probably deteriorated from the end of the first year, but this was not clinically apparent until 15–18 months later, when insulin doses were progressively increased.

(Table 2.2), and to non-specific macrovascular disease (coronary heart and peripheral vascular disease).

● Mortality in IDDM is increased 4- to 7-fold over the matched non-diabetic population; nephropathy and coronary heart disease are the main causes of death (Table 2.3).

● A proportion of IDDM patients survive without significant complications for many years; the factor(s) protecting them against complications are unknown.

Table 2.3. Causes of mortality in insulin-dependent (IDDM) and non-insulin-dependent (NIDDM) diabetes.

	IDDM (%)	NIDDM (%)
Cardiovascular disease	15	58
Cerebrovascular disease	3	12
Nephropathy	55	3
Diabetic 'coma'	4	1
Malignancy	0	11
Infections	10	4
Others	13	11

3: The clinical problem of non-insulin-dependent diabetes mellitus

- Non-insulin-dependent diabetes mellitus (NIDDM; Type 2) denotes diabetic patients who can survive long-term without insulin replacement, although many receive insulin to improve their glycaemic control.
- NIDDM affects about half a million people in the UK and comprises about 75% of the diabetic population (Table 3.1).
- Prevalence varies greatly between populations, being high in North American Indians and Micronesians of the Pacific and relatively low in the UK.
- Prevalence is high in migrant populations (e.g. Indians in South Africa, Trinidad, Singapore and the UK, Japanese in the USA).
- Prevalence is often higher in urban than in rural communities.
- It is uncertain whether the rising frequency in developed countries is explicable simply by the increasing proportion of older people in the population.
- Patients are mostly older and obese (Fig. 3.1) and present with insidious hyperglycaemic symptoms; many cases are diagnosed incidentally or because of the presence of diabetic complications (Table 3.2).
- NIDDM is apparently due to a combination of impaired insulin secretion (especially in non-obese subjects) and insensitivity of the target tissues to insulin (especially in obese subjects). There is a strong genetic predisposition to the disease.
- Specific microvascular complications are less common than in IDDM, where the onset is earlier and exposure to the disease generally longer. However, retinopathy (especially with maculopathy rather than proliferative changes), nephropathy (sometimes with renal failure) and neuropathy all occur.
- NIDDM carries a high risk of large-vessel atherosclerosis; commonly associated hypertension, hyperlipidaemia and obesity may contribute. Myocardial infarction is also common and accounts for 60% of deaths.
- NIDDM is not 'mild' diabetes: overall mortality is increased 2–3 fold and life expectancy reduced by 5–10 years.

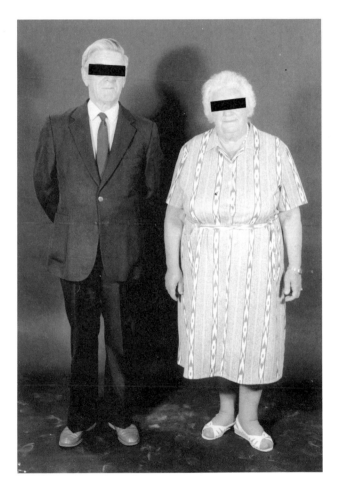

Fig. 3.1. The size of the problem: two distinct clinical subgroups of NIDDM, the non-obese and the obese. Aetiological factors differ, as does their management.

Table 3.1. Some important statistics concerning NIDDM.

• Very common	75% of all diabetic patients (500 000 in UK)
• Disease of ageing	Most patients >60 years
• Obesity common	Two-thirds are overweight
• Genetic factors important	40% have family history
• Male predominance	3:2 male excess

5

Table 3.2. Modes of presentation of NIDDM (UK Prospective Diabetes Study 1988).

Diabetic symptoms	53%
Incidental finding (usually glycosuria)	29%
Infections (e.g. candidiasis)	16%
Complications (e.g. retinopathy detected by an optician)	2%

Maturity-onset diabetes of the young (MODY)

● MODY is a variant of NIDDM currently best defined as hyperglycaemia diagnosed before 25 years of age and treatable for at least 5 years without insulin in patients who do not have immune or HLA markers of IDDM.
● MODY is rare in Caucasians, but commoner in Black races.
● MODY is generally inherited as an autosomal dominant gene.
● Many MODY families have low susceptibility to microvascular and/or macrovascular disease, but the syndrome shows considerable heterogeneity.
● Most newly-diagnosed young diabetic patients, even if of normal weight, will prove to have IDDM; all such patients should therefore be treated initially with insulin unless a strong family history suggests MODY.

4: The causes of insulin-dependent diabetes mellitus

Histology of the islet in IDDM

● In long-standing IDDM, all islets are insulin-deficient and devoid of B-cells, although A-, D- and PP-cells are preserved.
● In recent-onset IDDM, most islets are insulin-deficient, but the rest contain B-cells; some islets with residual B-cells show 'insulitis', i.e. infiltration with chronic inflammatory cells (see below), thought to be a manifestation of continuing and gradual autoimmune destruction (Fig. 4.1).

IDDM as an autoimmune disease

● Several lines of evidence suggest that humoral and cell-mediated autoimmune B-cell damage lead ultimately to IDDM.
● Circulating islet-cell antibodies (ICA) are found in most newly diagnosed IDDM patients (Fig. 4.2). ICA are class IgG and are directed against cytoplasmic antigens in B-cells and in the other islet endocrine cells. *In vitro*, ICA are cytotoxic to islet cells and impair insulin release but their *in vivo* actions are unknown.
● Spontaneous autoantibodies to insulin (IAA) also occur in many untreated, newly diagnosed IDDM patients.
● ICA and IAA are present during the prolonged 'prediabetic' period lasting up to several years before the clinical onset of IDDM, suggesting continuing autoimmune B-cell damage. Insulin secretion and glycaemia remain normal until relatively late in the disease process. After presentation, ICA and IAA titres generally fall progressively (Fig. 4.3).
● ICA also occur in close relatives of IDDM patients, especially in high-risk siblings who share one or both HLA haplotypes with the diabetic proband (Fig. 4.4). About 75% of those siblings with complement-fixing or high-titre (>20 JDF units) ICA will develop IDDM within 8 years. IAA may also predict susceptibility to IDDM.
● 'Insulitis' (the mononuclear cell infiltration of islets in newly diagnosed IDDM subjects) consists mainly of cytotoxic/suppressor T-lymphocytes and

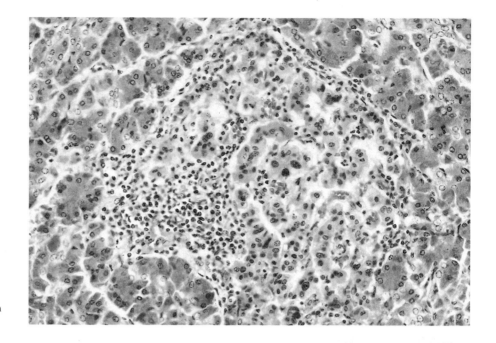

Fig. 4.1. Insulitis. There is a chronic inflammatory cell infiltrate centred on this islet. Haematoxylin and eosin stain (×300).

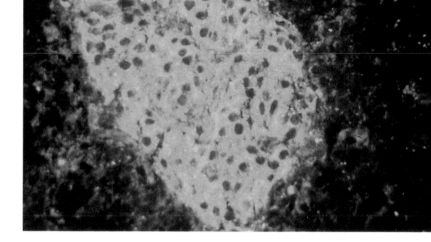

Fig. 4.2. Conventional islet cell antibodies (ICA). Cryostat section from a blood group O human pancreas stained by the indirect immunofluorescence technique. The section was first incubated with serum from an IDDM patient and subsequently stained with anti-human IgG fluoresceinated serum. All cells within the islet are strongly positive. The few orange granules scattered in the islet and in the exocrine portion of the gland are naturally occurring lipofuscin/lipid granules.

activated T-lymphocytes. The presence of these cells, together with penetration of IgG into islet B-cells and local complement deposition, strongly suggest an autoimmune process. Only islet B-cells are destroyed; the other islet endocrine cells remain intact (Fig. 4.5).

• Population studies show an association of IDDM with the HLA genes DR3 and DR4 (on chromosome 6) (Table 4.1). The maximum risk is for those who possess both DR3 and DR4 (14 times relative risk). In Japan, the association is with DR4/DRw9 and, in China, with DR3/DRw9.

• HLA class II antigens associated with an increased risk of IDDM (DR3, DR4) may optimize the presentation of islet B-cell autoantigens to T-helper lymphocytes and therefore promote autoimmune damage. By contrast, the HLA-DR2 molecule, which carries a reduced risk of IDDM, may have a configuration which impedes B-cell autoantigen presentation and therefore protects against autoimmune destruction.

• Cloning of the class II genes indicates that abnormalities of the DQβ molecule (lack of aspartate residue at position 57) might confer susceptibility to IDDM by altering the ability to present self-antigen to the immune system.

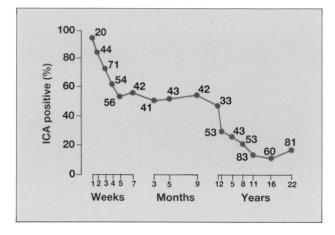

Fig. 4.3. Cross-sectional study showing a high prevalence of ICA at the time of diagnosis, but subsequently decreasing with time. Persistent ICA are found in approximately 10−15% of IDDM subjects. These cases tend to have similar clinical and immunological characteristics to patients with primary autoimmune endocrine disorders. The number of patients sampled at each point is indicated.

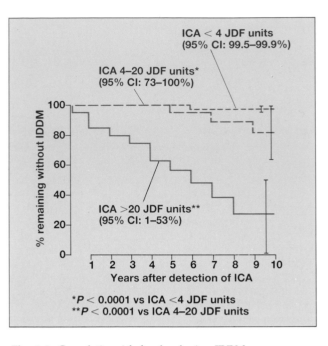

Fig. 4.4. Cumulative risk for developing IDDM over 10 years. The diagram summarizes the data on 719 first-degree relatives of IDDM probands in relation to peak titres of ICA level. The risk was greatest for relatives with the highest levels of ICA (>20 JDF units). 95% CI=95% confidence intervals.

- Cytokines released by activated lymphocytes and macrophages may enhance autoimmune damage, either by direct islet B-cell toxicity (e.g. interleukin-1) or by inducing aberrant expression or enhancing normal expression of HLA molecules by islet B-cells (e.g. interleukin-2).
- Viruses or other environmental agents may induce aberrant HLA class II antigen expression on islet B-cells which do not normally display these molecules. B-cells could then act as antigen-presenting cells, exposing their own surface antigen to T-helper lymphocytes (Fig. 4.6). Aberrant expression of class I antigens could similarly trigger cytotoxic T-lymphocyte activation. Both

mechanisms would lead to autoimmune B-cell destruction.

Viruses and environmental agents

- Involvement of viruses in causing human IDDM is suggested by epidemiological evidence, by the isolation of viruses from the pancreas and other tissues of a few recently diagnosed IDDM patients,

	Diabetic probands (*n*=122), % positive	Healthy subjects (*n*=110), % positive	Relative risk	95% confidence limits
DR2	4%	28%	0.1	0.05− 0.3
DR3	70%	32%	5.0	2.9 − 8.8
DR4	78%	34%	6.8	3.8 −12.1
DR3, DR4	51%	7%	14.3	6.3 −32.4
DR3, DRX	20%	25%	0.7	0.4 − 1.3
DR4, DRY	27%	27%	1.0	0.6 − 1.8
DRZ, DRZ	2.5%	50%	0.04	0.01− 0.13

Table 4.1. Relative risks associated with HLA-DR in IDDM subjects.

Data have been taken from Barts−Windsor Study.
DRX = any other antigen but DR4.
DRY = any other antigen but DR3.
DRZ = not DR3 or DR4.

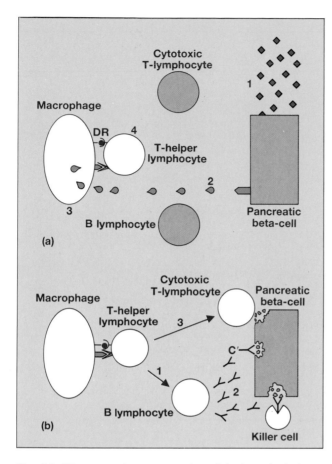

Fig. 4.5. Diagrammatic representation of the hypothetical steps leading to 'activation' of the immune system against the islet B-cell. In this scheme, the macrophage plays the central role in antigen presentation. (a) The triggering events: (1) Environmental attack (? viruses). (2) Release of autoantigens from the B-cell. (3) The macrophage processes the autoantigens and inserts them into its surface membrane. Class II molecules (DR) present islet autoantigens to the T-helper lymphocyte. (4) Activation of the T-helper lymphocyte. (b) Completing the vicious circle leading to death of the B-cell: (1) Activation of B-lymphocytes by the T-helper cell. (2) Production of islet-cell antibodies followed by antibody-dependent complement (C') and killer (K) cell-mediated cytoxicity. (3) Activation of the cytotoxic T-lymphocyte. (2) and (3) lead to lysis and death of the B-cell.
The T-suppressor lymphocyte is not represented in the diagram. The role of this cell in autoimmunity is not clearly understood at present but growing evidence indicates that organ B-cell-specific T-suppressor cells may exist, leading to de-repression of autoreactive helper and cytotoxic T-lymphocytes.

and by the ability of certain viruses to induce diabetes in animals (Table 4.2).
• Viruses may damage B-cells by direct invasion or by triggering an autoimmune response; they may also persist within B-cells, causing long-term interference with their metabolic and secretory functions.

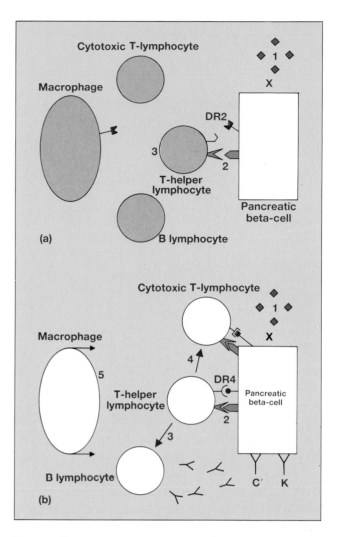

Fig. 4.6. Diagrammatic representation of the hypothetical steps leading to the 'activation' of the B-cell which in turn attracts immunocytes. In this scheme, the target B-cell plays the central role for antigen presentation. (a) *The 'wrong' presentation*: (1) Unknown environmental agents may stimulate class II molecule expression on the B-cell. (2) The phenomenon occurs in an HLA-DR2 individual who is protected against developing IDDM. (3) The T-helper cell is attracted, but the shape of the HLA-DR2 molecule is not 'ideal' to present the surface autoantigen on the B-cell. The interaction does not occur and the T-helper cell is not activated. (b) *The 'right' presentation*: (1) Similar initial events as described in (a). (2) The phenomenon leads to an aberrant expression of HLA-DR3 and/or DR4 molecules in a susceptible individual. The configuration of these particular class II products is now ideal to present the surface autoantigen on the B-cell. The T-helper cell recognizes the complex and becomes activated. (3) The B-lymphocyte is activated and produces islet-cell antibodies. Cytotoxicity follows via C'- and K-cell activation. (4) The signal is also sent to the cytotoxic T-lymphocyte which is attracted by the enhanced expression of HLA class I molecules on the B-cells. (5) The macrophage obeys its physiological function and it finally moves in to clear the cellular debris.

Table 4.2. Viruses implicated in the development of insulin-dependent diabetes.

Virus	Family	Nucleic acid	In vivo	In vitro
Coxsackie B1	Picornaviridae	RNA	Man, mouse	
Coxsackie B2	Picornaviridae	RNA	Man, mouse	
Coxsackie B3	Picornaviridae	RNA	Mouse, monkey	Human B-cells
Coxsackie B4	Picornaviridae	RNA	Man[‡], mouse, monkey	Human B-cells, human islets
Coxsackie B5	Picornaviridae	RNA	Man[†], mouse	
Coxsackie B6	Picornaviridae	RNA	Man, mouse	
Echovirus 4	Picornaviridae	RNA	Man	
Encephalomyocarditis	Picornaviridae	RNA	Mouse	Mouse islets, mouse B-cells
Foot-and-mouth disease	Picornaviridae	RNA	Pig, cow	
Poliovirus	Picornaviridae	RNA	Man	
Mengovirus	Picornaviridae	RNA	Mouse	
Mumps	Paramyxoviridae	RNA	Man	Human B-cells, monkey B-cells
Rubella	Togaviridae	RNA	Man[*†], hamster, rabbit	
Tick-borne encephalitis	Togaviridae	RNA	Man	
Venezuelan equine encephalitis	Togaviridae	RNA	Monkey, hamster, mouse	
Infectious hepatitis	Pararetroviridae	RNA	Man	
Reovirus	Reoviridae	RNA	Mouse	Human B-cells
Influenza	Orthomyxoviridae	RNA	Man	
Cytomegalovirus	Herpesviridae	DNA	Man[*†]	Human islets
Herpes virus 6	Herpesviridae	DNA	Man	
Epstein–Barr virus	Herpesviridae	DNA	Man	
Varicella zoster	Herpesviridae	DNA	Man	
Scrapie agent	?	?	Hamster	
Lymphocytic choriomeningitic virus	Arenaviridae	DNA	Mouse	

[*] Intrauterine infection. [†] Virus isolated from tissues. [‡] Virus isolated from pancreas.

• Mumps virus can cause acute pancreatitis, sometimes with hyperglycaemia, but serological and epidemiological evidence implicating mumps infection in IDDM patients is equivocal.

• *Intrauterine* rubella infection is definitely associated with subsequent development of IDDM; the virus may persist within T-cells and predispose to autoimmune disease. *Postnatal* rubella can stimulate islet-cell and insulin autoantibody formation but does not apparently lead to IDDM.

• Coxsackie B viruses (especially B4) can cause acute pancreatitis and B-cell destruction in man; although usually tropic for pancreatic exocrine tissue, certain strains become able to invade B-cells. Some (but not all) serological studies suggest an increased frequency of previous exposure to the virus in newly diagnosed IDDM patients. Coxsackie B viruses have been isolated from acute cases of IDDM and some of these are diabetogenic in animals.

• Other viruses implicated in human IDDM include echoviruses, cytomegalovirus and herpes viruses.

• Vacor is a rodenticide which is B-cell cytoxic and has caused IDDM following ingestion by man. Dietary nitrosamines (present in some smoked meats) may also be diabetogenic in man and animals.

Clues from animal models of IDDM

• Insulin-deficient diabetes can be induced in animals by administration of a number of chemicals, principally alloxan, streptozotocin and zinc chelators (Table 4.3).

• Alloxan may act at several sites in the B-cell, such as on glucose transporters on the cell surface, and intracellularly on the sulphydryl groups of glucokinase, and on the mitochondria by inducing free radical formation, and by inducing DNA strand breaks. DNA damage stimulates DNA repair by poly(ADP-ribose) synthetase and leads to cellular NAD depletion (Fig. 4.7).

• Streptozotocin in a single large dose probably has similar effects to alloxan, including DNA damage and free radical generation. It also causes diabetes after repeated injection of subdiabetogenic doses into genetically susceptible mice,

Table 4.3. Chemical diabetogenic agents.

	Zinc chelator (8-hydroxyquinoline)	Alloxan	Streptozotocin
Name	hydroxybenzopyridine	2,4,5,6-tetraoxohexa-hydropyrimidine	2-deoxy-2-[((methyl-nitrosoamino) carbonyl)-amino]-D-glucopyranose
Structure			
Therapeutic use	Fungistatic Disinfectant	Antineoplastic agent	Antineoplastic agent Antibiotic
Diabetogenic effects	Permanent diabetes No B-cell lysis No insulitis	Permanent diabetes Direct B-cell cytotoxicity Necrosis but *no* insulitis	Permanent diabetes Direct B-cell cytotoxicity Insulitis at low doses

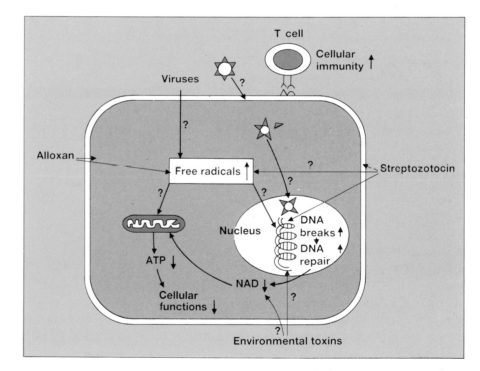

Fig. 4.7. Effects of environmental factors on the pancreatic B-cell. Viruses and other environmental agents may either activate cellular HLA class I and II expression on the B-cell, or produce a variety of biochemical effects on and in the B-cell, including DNA strand breaks and consequent NAD depletion, and actions on the mitochondrion, glucokinase and glucose transporters. Some of these effects may be mediated by free radical production.

where there is pancreatic insulitis and an immune mechanism is implicated.

● Spontaneous diabetes occurs in the BB rat and the NOD mouse, which are the best available models of human IDDM (Table 4.4).

● The BB rat is characterized by a genetic predisposition to IDDM. This occurs after a long prediabetic period and is associated with hypoinsulinaemia, ketoacidosis and a mononuclear cell infiltrate of the islets which precedes the overt hyperglycaemia.

● Defects in cellular and humoral immunity are involved in diabetes in the BB rat, e.g. the presence of islet-cell-surface antibodies in diabetes-prone and newly diabetic animals and destruction of normal rat islets by splenic lymphoid cells from BB rats. Diabetes may be prevented by many immunomodulatory procedures such as cyclosporin-A, antilymphocyte serum treatment and neonatal thymectomy.

● Diabetes in the NOD mouse is similar to that in the BB rat (e.g. insulitis preceding the hyperglycaemia) but only 80% of females and 20% of males are affected.

Characteristic	Man	BB rat	NOD mouse
MHC association	Yes	Yes	Yes
Long prediabetic period	Yes	Yes	Yes
Insulitis	Yes	Yes	Yes
Insulin-dependent/ketosis-prone	Yes	Yes	Yes
Obese	No	No	No
Sex difference	No	No	♀ > ♂
ICA/ICSA	Yes/yes	No/yes	Yes/yes
64kDa islet-cell protein antibodies[†]	Yes	Yes	Yes
Other autoantibodies (thyroid, lymphocyte)	Yes	Yes	Yes
Lymphopenia	No	Yes*	Yes
Functional T-cell defects	No	Yes*	Yes
Thyroiditis	Yes	Yes	Yes
Role of environmental agents	Yes	Yes	Yes

Table 4.4. Characteristics of IDDM in man, and in the animal models of IDDM, the BB rat and NOD mouse.

* Not in all BB rat colonies. [†] Antibodies are directed against a protein of molecular weight 64 000. The protein is therefore termed the '64 Da' antigen; recent evidence suggests that it may be the enzyme glutamate decarboxylase.
MHC = major histocompatibility complex. ICA/ICSA = islet-cell/islet-cell-surface antibodies.

5: The causes of non-insulin-dependent diabetes mellitus

Histology of islets in NIDDM

• Total islet and B-cell mass are reduced to 50–60% of normal in NIDDM.
• The mass of the glucagon-producing A-cells is increased.
• The most important morphological feature is amyloid deposition in the islets (Fig. 5.1). These deposits consist of islet amyloid polypeptide (IAPP or amylin).
• IAPP has 50% homology with the regulatory peptide, calcitonin-gene-related peptide (CGRP) and there is evidence that it originates in the B-cell secretory granules.

Insulin resistance

• The biological response to insulin is reduced (by about 40%) in NIDDM, as shown by studies with the euglycaemic clamp, insulin tolerance tests and mathematical modelling of i.v. glucose tolerance tests (Fig. 5.2).
• Insulin resistance in NIDDM involves effects on both hepatic glucose output and peripheral glucose uptake.
• Hyperglycaemia itself causes insulin resistance and impaired insulin secretion ('glucose toxicity') but many factors also contribute to the insensitivity, including obesity, age, lack of exercise, diet and genetic components.
• The mechanisms of insulin resistance in NIDDM are unclear but may involve reduced insulin receptor numbers (secondary to hyperinsulinaemia and hyperglycaemia), reduced tyrosine kinase activity of the insulin receptor and abnormalities distal to the receptor.

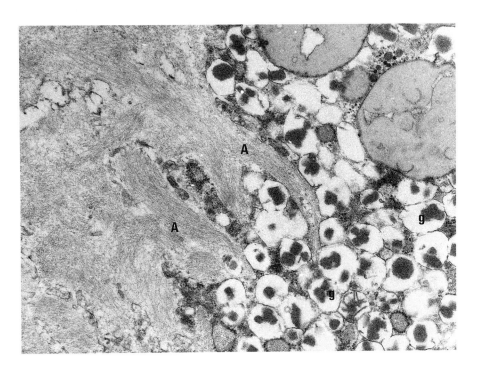

Fig. 5.1. Electron micrograph of islet amyloid adjacent to a B-cell which contains many secretory, insulin-containing granules (g). The amyloid fibrils (A) are arranged in bundles running into deep pockets in the cell membrane. This appearance is not seen when the amyloid occurs close to other islet cells and is interpreted as a sign of fibril production by the B-cells.

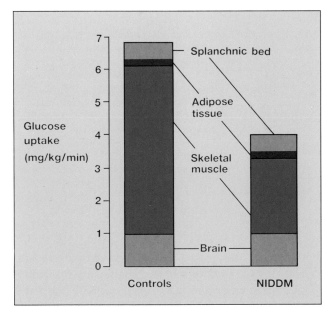

Fig. 5.2. Insulin resistance in NIDDM as shown by the reduced glucose uptake in various tissues as compared with non-diabetic subjects, under conditions of elevated insulin levels (euglycaemic clamp). Note the major contribution of muscle to insulin resistance.

Abnormalities of pancreatic insulin secretion

• In early NIDDM, the absolute basal insulin levels are normal or elevated, but inappropriately low in comparison with the raised blood glucose concentrations. Moreover, recent studies suggest that much of the 'insulin' measured by conventional assays is in fact abnormal cleavage products of proinsulin; most NIDDM patients probably have absolute insulin deficiency. The pulsatility of basal insulin secretion is abnormal in NIDDM, possibly making the insulin less biologically effective.

• The first phase of insulin secretion in response to glucose is deficient in NIDDM (see Fig. 5.3), causing post-prandial hyperglycaemia through insulin deficiency and the lack of the priming effect of the first-phase insulin on the target organs. The response to non-glucose stimuli is normal, suggesting a specific glucoreceptor abnormality (Fig. 5.3).

• With persistent hyperglycaemia, the second phase of insulin release in response to glucose becomes attenuated in NIDDM.

• There is a 'horseshoe-shaped' relationship between the insulin response and the plasma glucose level in NIDDM. Insulin secretion increases progressively as the glucose level increases to about 7 mmol/l, after which further increases cause a decline in insulin secretion. This may indicate a toxic effect of hyperglycaemia on the B-cells. This relationship has been termed 'starling's curve' of the pancreas (Fig. 5.4).

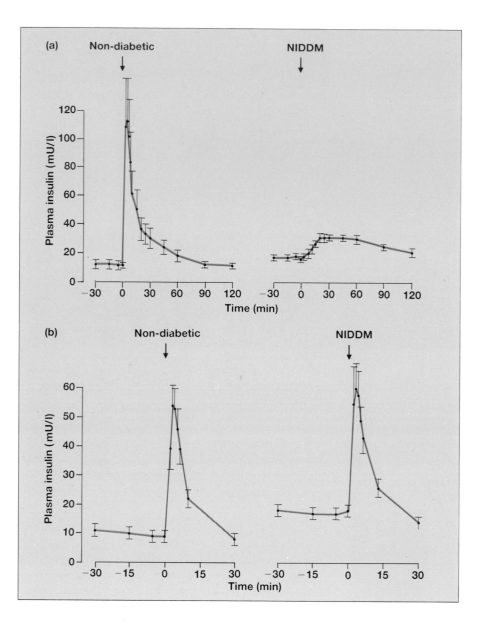

Fig. 5.3. (a) Mean ± SEM plasma insulin concentrations in non-diabetic subjects and NIDDM patients after 20 g glucose given intravenously (arrow). Note lack of first-phase insulin response and relatively well-preserved second-phase response in NIDDM. (b) Mean ± SEM plasma insulin in non-diabetic subjects and NIDDM patients in response to intravenous arginine (arrow). Note normal response in NIDDM to this non-glucose stimulant, indicating a specific glucoreceptor abnormality.

Obesity as a risk factor for NIDDM

- NIDDM is strongly associated with obesity (Fig. 5.5); the risks of developing NIDDM increase progressively with rising body-mass index, with an added risk from a high waist/hip ratio indicating central fat deposition. Insulin resistance associated with obesity may demand excessive insulin secretion and contribute to B-cell exhaustion.
- The tendency to obesity is partly inherited but its development depends on environmental factors such as food availability and cultural influences.
- A central body fat distribution, with a high waist/hip ratio and an 'android' or 'apple-shaped' habitus, is associated with insulin resistance, NIDDM, hyperlipidaemia and premature mortality (Fig. 5.6). A peripheral ('gynoid' or 'pear-shaped') distribution with a lower waist/hip ratio is found in individuals who exercise and do not carry these disease associations.
- A Western-style, high-fat, low-carbohydrate, low-fibre diet predisposes to obesity and is associated with NIDDM; the dietary risk factors responsible have complex interactions with each other.
- Dietary sugar does not alone cause obesity or NIDDM but in large amounts can aggravate hyperglycaemia in decompensated diabetes.
- Exercise may protect against NIDDM as well as increasing energy expenditure and so opposing weight gain.

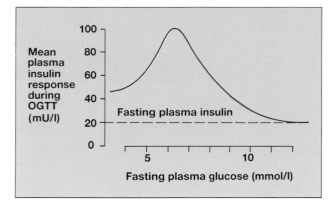

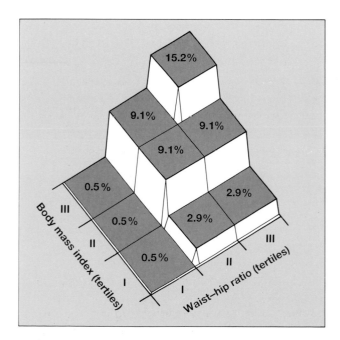

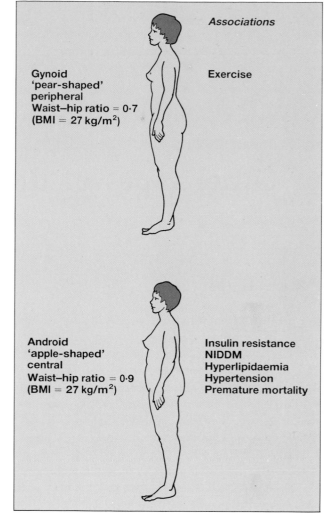

Fig. 5.4. 'Starling's curve' of the pancreas. In normal-weight patients with impaired glucose tolerance and mild diabetes mellitus, plasma insulin response to ingested glucose increases progressively until the fasting glucose concentration reaches about 6.7 mmol/l. Thereafter, further increases in fasting glucose level are associated with a progressive decline in insulin secretion, perhaps indicating a toxic effect of glucose on B-cell function. The same curve depicts the relationship between fasting plasma insulin and glucose concentration.

Fig. 5.5. Predictive values of BMI and WHR for the development of NIDDM. BMI and WHR were classified into tertiles (I = lowest, III = greatest) in a population of middle-aged Swedish men. The risk of developing diabetes during the 13-year study period is shown on top of each bar. BMI = body mass index: Weight in kg/(height in m)²; WHR = waist/hip ratio.

Fig. 5.6. The extremes of body fat distribution and their main metabolic associations. NIDDM is strongly associated with obesity, particularly when centrally distributed. Insulin resistance may contribute to B-cell exhaustion by causing excessive insulin secretion.

Genetics of NIDDM

● An important genetic contribution to NIDDM is suggested by the very high concordance rates of the disease in monozygotic, genetically identical twins. Many of the apparently unaffected co-twins of the diabetic twins have subclinical defects in insulin secretion, sometimes with mild hyperglycaemia. Dizygotic, non-identical twins show much lower concordance rates.

● The inheritance of NIDDM is apparently polygenic in most pedigrees. However, maturity-onset diabetes of the young (MODY) is transmitted as an autosomal dominant gene and various rare syndromes which include glucose intolerance and/or NIDDM are inherited by classical Mendelian patterns.

● Molecular biological techniques have identified the molecular lesions in certain cases of insulinopathy and of inherited insulin receptor abnormalities which cause rare NIDDM-like syndromes.

• In contrast to IDDM, there are no strong associations between NIDDM and HLA type in Caucasian populations. However, certain associations with HLA status have been discovered in other races, notably the complement component, C4B (an HLA class III antigen), in South Indian subjects and Bw 61 in South African Indians.

6: Other types of diabetes

Pancreatic disease

• Chronic pancreatitis, due especially to alcohol abuse in Western countries, is complicated by diabetes in about 30% of cases with non-calcific and 70% of those with calcific disease (Fig. 6.1). Ketoacidosis is rare but one-third of cases require insulin; insulin-related hypoglycaemia may be severe. Abstention from alcohol is crucial and pancreatic enzyme supplements should be prescribed.

• Glucose intolerance occurs in 30% of patients with cystic fibrosis; overt diabetes develops in 1–2% of affected children and in up to 13% of patients surviving beyond the age of 25 years.

• Diabetes with variable insulin resistance and sometimes accompanied by microvascular com-

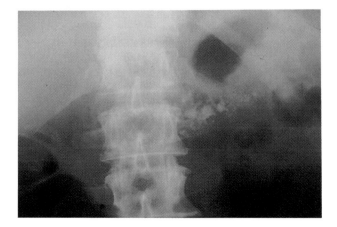

Fig. 6.1. Plain abdominal radiograph showing pancreatic calcification due to chronic pancreatitis, a condition often associated with diabetes.

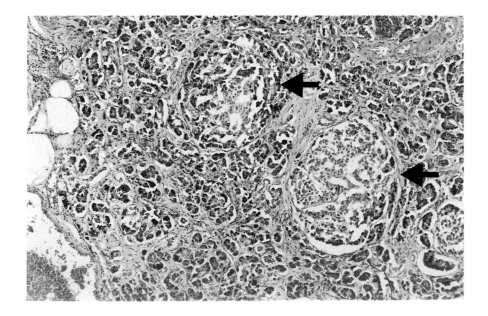

Fig. 6.2. Section of pancreas from a patient with haemochromatosis, showing heavy deposition of iron (stained blue) in acinar tissue and islets (arrows). Perl's stain. 50–60% of patients with haemochromatosis develop diabetes.

plications develops in 50—60% of patients with haemochromatosis (Fig. 6.2). Effective reduction of the iron overload may improve glucose tolerance and lower insulin requirements.
• Totally pancreatectomized subjects develop IDDM and are susceptible to ketoacidosis and to microvascular complications. Because of the lack of pancreatic glucagon counter-regulation, insulin replacement frequently causes severe and prolonged hypoglycaemia.

Endocrinopathies

• Impaired glucose tolerance (IGT) and overt diabetes each affect up to 30% of acromegalic patients, and improve with effective treatment of the acromegaly (Fig. 6.3). The development of growth hormone deficiency in insulin-treated diabetic patients can lead to severe hypoglycaemia.
• Hyperthyroidism causes mild glucose intolerance (reversible with anti-thyroid treatment) and can worsen metabolic control in diabetic patients.
• IDDM affects about 10% of patients with Addison's disease; diabetic patients who develop Addison's disease become increasingly insulin-sensitive and suffer frequent hypoglycaemia.
• Diabetes (usually non-ketotic) affects about 25% of patients with Cushing's syndrome and resolves with effective treatment (Fig. 6.4). Glucocorticoids stimulate hepatic gluconeogenesis and inhibit glucose uptake into peripheral tissues.
• About 50% of patients with Conn's syndrome have glucose intolerance and a few have NIDDM; potassium depletion apparently impairs insulin secretion.
• Up to 75% of phaeochromocytoma patients have glucose intolerance, attributed to catecholamine-mediated increases in hepatic glycogen breakdown and to inhibition of insulin secretion.
• Mild, non-ketotic diabetes is a feature of the very rare glucagonoma (Table 6.1, Fig. 6.5), somatostatinoma and VIPoma syndromes.

Table 6.1. Clinical features of the glucagonoma syndrome.

Necrolytic migratory erythematous rash
Angular stomatis and glossitis
Mild diabetes mellitus, usually without ketosis
Weight loss and muscle wasting
Normochromic normocytic anaemia
Hypoaminoacidaemia
Thromboembolism
Neuropsychiatric disturbances

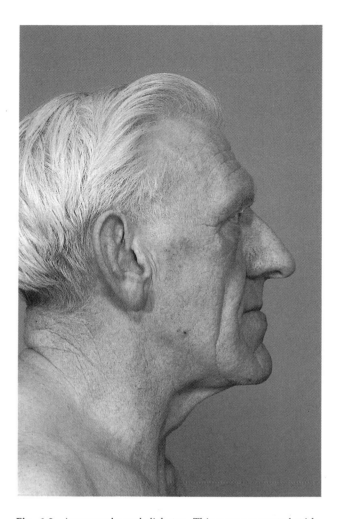

Fig. 6.3. Acromegaly and diabetes. This man presented with thirst and polyuria and was found to have a fasting blood glucose concentration of 11 mmol/l. Further questioning revealed a 15-year history of acral enlargement, sweating and headache. Growth hormone levels were moderately high (30—40 mU/l) during hyperglycaemia. Computerized tomography (CT) scanning demonstrated a large pituitary adenoma which was successfully removed by the transphenoidal route. Postoperatively, he has remained normoglycaemic.

Insulinopathies

• Insulinopathies arise from rare mutations in the human insulin gene which lead to the synthesis and secretion of abnormal gene products (Table 6.2).
• Such patients usually display hyperinsulinaemia, varying degrees of glucose intolerance (sometimes normal) and a normal response to exogenous insulin administration. The defect is inherited in an autosomal fashion with all subjects to date being heterozygous for the normal and mutant alleles.

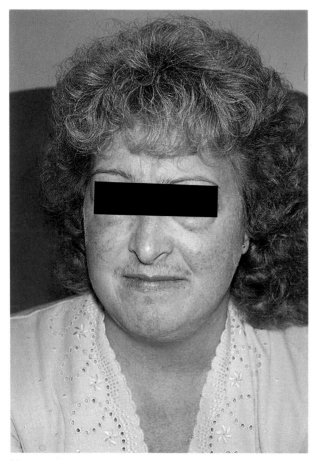

(a)

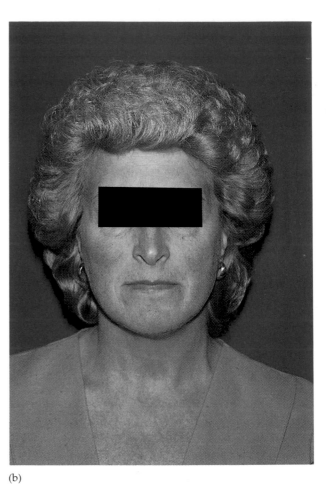

(b)

Fig. 6.4. This 43-year-old woman was referred to the diabetic clinic with glycosuria. Oral glucose tolerance testing revealed IGT. Cushing's syndrome, suggested by her rounded, plethoric face and facial hirsutes (a) and truncal obesity, was diagnosed and successfully treated by transphenoidal removal of a pituitary microadenoma. Postoperatively, her Cushingoid features resolved (b) and a repeat glucose tolerance test was normal.

- Sophisticated techniques of peptide chemistry and DNA analysis have shown single nucleotide changes resulting in an amino-acid replacement and either an abnormal insulin of similar molecular weight to native insulin, or interference with the processing of proinsulin to insulin (e.g. C-peptide remaining joined at the insulin A chain—Table 6.3).

- Subjects with insulinopathy and diabetes may have additional abnormalities in, for example, the insulin secretion process or at the receptor site.

Insulin resistance

- Insulin resistance (with hyperinsulinaemia and

Table 6.2. Clinical findings in insulinopathies associated with diabetes.

Abnormal findings	Normal findings
Elevated level of serum immunoreactive insulin	Normal levels of monocyte insulin receptors
Elevated serum insulin: C-peptide molar ratio	Normal levels of counter-regulatory (anti-insulin) hormones
Mild to severe glucose intolerance	Normal response to administered insulin

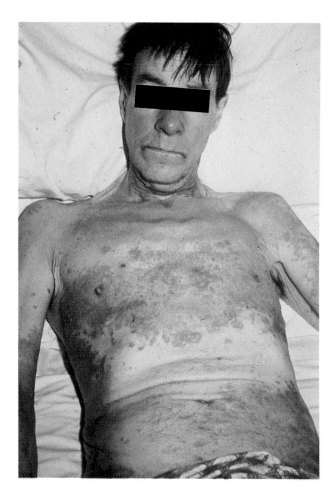

Fig. 6.5. Necrolytic migratory erythema characteristic of the glucagonoma syndrome. This patient had recurrent episodes of the rash together with non-ketotic diabetes which was easily controlled with low dosages of insulin. Despite his increasingly cachectic appearance and several large hepatic metastases, he survived for over 5 years before dying of massive pulmonary embolism.

various degrees of hyperglycaemia) is associated with several rare syndromes, either congenital or acquired, including acanthosis nigricans, 'leprechaunism' and lipoatrophy (Table 6.4).

• Insulin resistance with acanthosis nigricans is subdivided into 'Type A' (hereditary) and 'Type B' (autoimmune) syndromes (Fig. 6.6).

• The Type A syndrome, due to various genetic defects in the insulin receptor, predominantly affects young women who are grossly hyper-insulinaemic, markedly glucose-intolerant and usually virilized. Type A variants (including the 'Type C' syndrome) are clinically similar but due to a *post*receptor defect.

• The Type B syndrome, due to antibodies (usually IgG) directed against the insulin receptor, also mainly affects women who often have other features of generalized autoimmune disease. Most patients are hyperglycaemic but specific receptor-*stimulating* antibodies in a few may cause hypo-glycaemia. Type B variants include other rare conditions with anti-insulin-receptor antibodies (e.g. ataxia telangiectasia).

• 'Leprechaunism' is a rare and fatal congenital syndrome of extreme insulin resistance due to in-herited defects of the insulin receptor. Associated growth retardation and multiple somatic abnor-malities may be due to coexistent resistance to other growth factors.

• Lipoatrophy may be congenital or acquired and is characterized by loss of subcutaneous fat, which may be either partial or generalized (Fig. 6.7). Growth disturbances, hepatomegaly and gross hypertriglyceridaemia are associated with certain

Table 6.3. Known examples of mutant human insulin genes and associated abnormal insulins.

Name	Amino acid replacement	Designation	Normal codon	Mutant codon	Abnormal secreted product
Insulin Chicago	Phe^{B25} by Leu	Human insulin B25 (Phe → Leu)	TTC	TTG	[Leu^{B25}] insulin*
Insulin Los Angeles	Phe^{B24} by Ser	Human insulin B24 (Phe → Ser)	TTC	TCC	[Ser^{B24}] insulin*
Insulin Wakayama	Val^{A3} by Leu	Human insulin A3 (Val → Leu)	GTG	TTG	[Leu^{A3}] insulin*
Proinsulin Tokyo	Arg^{65} by His	Human proinsulin 65 (Arg → His)	CGC	CAC	des-Arg^{31}, Arg^{32}-[His^{65}] proinsulin†
Proinsulin Boston‡	Arg^{65} by ?	Human proinsulin 65 (Arg →?)‡	?	?	des-Arg^{31}, Arg^{32}-[Xxx] proinsulin
Proinsulin Providence	His^{B10} by Asp	Human proinsulin 10 (His → Asp)	CAC	GAC	?§

* The secreted product is an abnormal insulin which contains a single amino acid replacement.
† The secreted product is an abnormal intermediate of proinsulin processing in which the C peptide remains joined to the insulin A chain due to an amino acid replacement at the processing site.
‡ The gene for Proinsulin Boston has not yet been subjected to sequence analysis. The nature of the secreted product is the same as that for Proinsulin Tokyo, but the amino acid replacement is not yet known.
§ The exact structures of the secreted products are not known. They appear, for the most part, to represent intact proinsulin (rather than insulin or a processing intermediate), but they have not yet been analysed in detail.

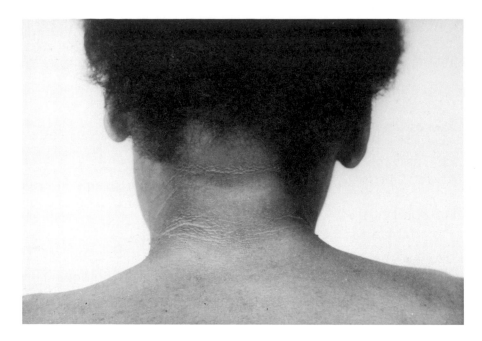

Fig. 6.6. Acanthosis nigricans. Typical appearance of papillomatosis and hyperpigmentation on the neck of an individual with severe insulin resistance.

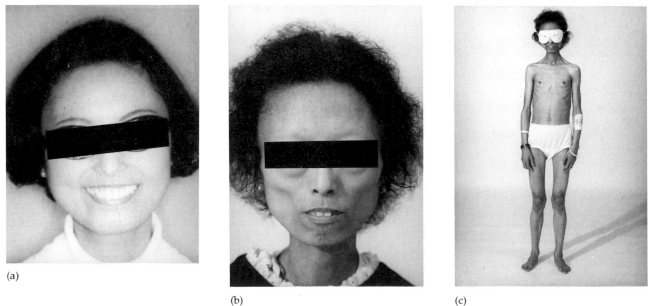

(a)

(b)

(c)

Fig. 6.7. Acquired, generalized (total) lipoatrophy. (a) Appearance of patient before onset of lipoatrophy. (b) Facial features of patient showing dramatic loss of subcutaneous adipose tissue. (c) Generalized loss of body fat in frontal view. Insulin resistance and diabetes due to receptor or post-receptor defects are features of this condition.

Table 6.4. Syndromes of insulin resistance with acanthosis nigricans. (+) Present, (−) not present.

	Type A	Type B	Generalized lipoatrophy	Leprechaunism
Clinical features				
Peak age of onset (years)	10−20	30−60	10−20	0−1
Acromegaloid features	+	−	+	−
Hirsutism	+	+	+	+
Polycystic ovaries and virilization	+	+	+	+
Hepatomegaly	−	−	+	+
Laboratory findings				
Anti-insulin-receptor antibodies	−	+++	−	−
Antinuclear antibodies	−	+	−	−
Hyperlipidaemia	−	−	+++	+
Hyperandrogenaemia	+	+	+	+
Fasting hypoglycaemia	−	+/−	−	++
Insulin resistance in cultured cells	+++	−	+/−	+++

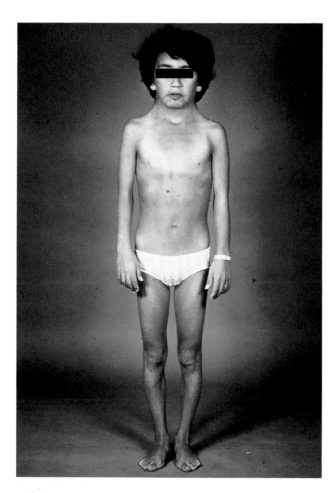

Fig. 6.8. A 15-year-old patient with Turner's disease showing short stature, webbed neck and broad chest with widely spaced nipples. Two-thirds of such patients may develop diabetes or IGT.

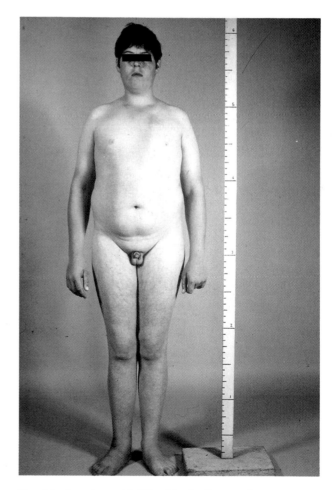

Fig. 6.9. A patient with Klinefelter's disease, showing increased height with eunuchoid build, gynaecomastia and underdeveloped genitalia. One-quarter of such patients may develop diabetes or IGT.

forms. Severe insulin resistance and diabetes (often presenting in the teens) may be due to receptor or postreceptor defects.

Genetic disorders associated with diabetes

- Several syndromes of inherited insulin resistance are associated with diabetes, including Alström's, Laurence—Moon—Biedl, Prader—Willi and Rabson—Mendenhall syndromes, and dystrophia myotonica (Table 6.5).
- Diabetes, often insulin-requiring, affects up to 2% of children with Down's syndrome.
- Two-thirds of women with Turner's syndrome have a diabetic oral glucose tolerance curve although symptomatic diabetes is rare (Fig. 6.8).
- One-quarter of men with Klinefelter's syndrome have mild insulin resistance and a diabetic oral glucose tolerance curve; overt diabetes affects fewer than 10% (Fig. 6.9).
- Impaired glucose tolerance (IGT) and occasionally diabetes may complicate acute intermittent porphyria, in which attacks may be provoked by chlorpropamide, tolbutamide and tolazamide. Biguanides, glipizide and insulin can be used safely in acute intermittent porphyria.
- The prevalence of diabetes in adults with coeliac disease is 4%, some 2—3 times higher than in the general population. Hypoglycaemia may be troublesome, especially during exacerbations of diarrhoea. A gluten-free diet may increase insulin requirements.

Table 6.5. Classification of genetic disorders associated with increased prevalence of diabetes mellitus.

CHROMOSOMAL DEFECTS
Down's syndrome (trisomy or translocation 21)
Turner's syndrome (45,XO or variants)
Klinefelter's syndrome (47,XXY)

SINGLE-GENE DEFECTS
Pancreatic disorders
Cystic fibrosis (autosomal recessive)
Haemochromatosis (autosomal dominant)

Inborn errors of metabolism
Acute intermittent porphyria

Inherited insulin resistance syndromes
Group I (with hypogonadism):
 Alström's syndrome (autosomal recessive)
 Laurence—Moon—Biedl syndrome (autosomal recessive)
 Prader—Willi syndrome (deletion/translocation chromosome 15)
 Werner's syndrome (autosomal recessive)
 Cockayne's syndrome (autosomal recessive)
 Ataxia telangiectasia (autosomal recessive)
 Dystrophia myotonica (autosomal dominant)
Group II (with sexual precocity):
 Rabson—Mendenhall syndrome (autosomal recessive)
 Leprechaunism (autosomal recessive)
 Lipodystrophic syndromes (various inheritance patterns)

Miscellaneous endocrine syndromes
Type II polyglandular autoimmune syndrome (Schmidt's syndrome) (autosomal dominant or recessive in some pedigrees)
DIDMOAD (Wolfram's syndrome) (autosomal recessive)
Friedreich's ataxia (autosomal recessive)
Huntington's chorea (autosomal dominant)

7: Diabetic control and its management

- The presence or absence of glycosuria may be highly misleading even in diabetic patients with a normal threshold for glucose reabsorption, and urinary glucose measurements do not warn of hypoglycaemia. Testing for glycosuria is therefore a very unsatisfactory means of assessing glycaemic control.

- Single blood glucose measurements are a poor guide to overall glycaemic control in IDDM patients, but fasting or postprandial levels correlate significantly with glycated haemoglobin (HbA$_1$) levels in NIDDM and may therefore be used to monitor control in these patients.
- The use of 'dry chemistry' reagent test strips

(based on glucose oxidase) to measure blood glucose concentrations has revolutionized self-monitoring of diabetic control by the patient. This is discussed in detail on p. 29.

• Glycated (or glycosylated) haemoglobin comprises a series of minor haemoglobin components (HbA$_{1a}$, HbA$_{1b}$ and HbA$_{1c}$) formed by the non-enzymatic adduction of glucose and glucose-derived products to normal adult haemoglobin (HbA$_0$). The steps in the reaction which leads the formation of a stable ketoamine derivative are shown in Fig. 7.1.

• The level of HbA$_1$ (expressed as a percentage of total HbA) reflects the integrated glycaemic level (Fig. 7.2), and therefore the mean blood glucose concentration over the preceding 6–8 weeks (i.e. the half-life of the red cell).

• HbA$_1$ can be measured by several methods; affinity chromatography is most widely used and is not affected by the presence of the labile component of HbA$_1$ (which is unrelated to long-term

glycaemic levels) or by haemoglobinopathy.

• Target ranges for HbA$_1$ depend on the assay and the laboratory; the non-diabetic range is usually about 5–9%. Nearly normal HbA$_1$ values are more easily obtained in NIDDM or C-peptide-positive IDDM patients early in the course of their disease.

• HbA$_1$ values may be spuriously lowered by reduced red cell survival (e.g. bleeding or haemo-

Table 7.1. Factors affecting glycosylated haemoglobin assays.

Spuriously low HbA$_1$	Spuriously high HbA$_1$
Reduced red-cell survival (blood loss, haemolysis)	Carbamylated HbA$_0$ (in uraemia)
Haemoglobinopathy: HbS and/or HbC	Haemoglobinopathy (HbF)

Note: affinity chromatography is not affected by abnormal haemoglobins.

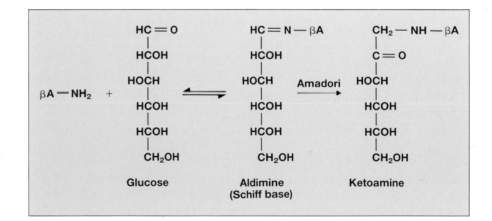

Fig. 7.1. Schematic representation of the adduction of glucose to the terminal valine of the B chain of HbA to form HbA$_{1c}$. The unstable aldimine intermediate (a Schiff base) undergoes an 'Amadori rearrangement' to form the final, stable ketoamine derivative.

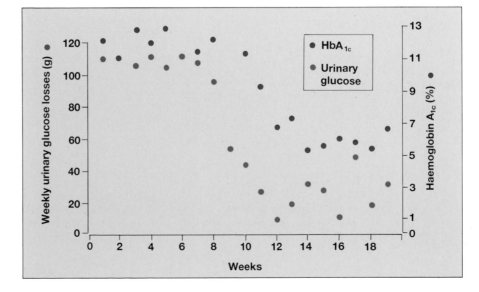

Fig. 7.2. Changes in HbA$_{1c}$ and urinary glucose in a diabetic patient when glycaemic control was improved from week 7 onwards. Note the delay in HbA$_{1c}$ reduction compared with urinary glucose levels.

lysis) and by slowly migrating haemoglobins (HbS and/or HbC), and falsely raised by rapidly migrating haemoglobins (HbF, or the carbamylated HbA occurring in uraemia) (Table 7.1).

• Glycated serum proteins (notably albumin, measured by the 'fructosamine' reaction) turn over more rapidly than haemoglobin and provide a measure of short-term (7–14 days) integrated glycaemic control.

• Fructosamine assays are cheap and simple to perform but levels fluctuate widely in diabetic patients due to variations in serum protein concentrations, and are also affected by uraemia and other conditions. Fructosamine measurements are not a substitute for the more expensive HbA_1 estimations and their place in routine diabetic management remains controversial.

8: The metabolic importance of endogenous B-cell function and C peptide

• Peripheral insulin levels cannot be used to assess B-cell function because of large and variable uptake from the portal circulation into the liver, and because insulin assays cannot distinguish endogenous from exogenous insulin.

• C peptide is a marker for B-cell function because it is secreted in equimolar amounts to insulin of proinsulin following proteolytic cleavage (Fig. 8.1). This cleavage process may be abnormal in NIDDM, leading to the secretion of large amounts of proinsulin 'split products' which are biologically less active, but cross-react in conventional assays for insulin.

• Circulating C-peptide concentrations may be a more stable index of B-cell function than insulin as the former is only minimally extracted by the liver (Fig. 8.2).

• The best established measures of B-cell function are the plasma C-peptide responses to a standard meal (e.g. 'Sustacal') or the intravenous injection of glucagon.

• Even minimally preserved B-cell function is metabolically beneficial, being associated with lower insulin dosages, lower HbA_{1c} levels and less metabolic decompensation after insulin withdrawal (Fig. 8.3).

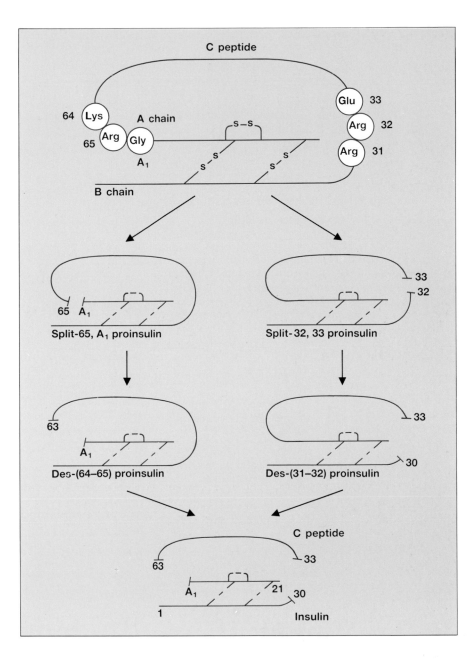

Fig. 8.1. Processing of proinsulin to insulin in the secretory granules of the B cell involves proteolytic cleavage of proinsulin, producing equimolar amounts of a connecting peptide (C peptide) and insulin. C-peptide levels in the peripheral circulation can be used as a marker of remaining B-cell function in diabetic patients.

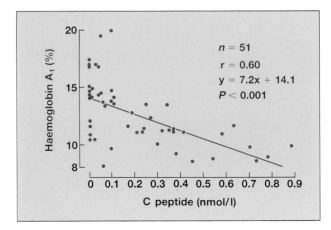

Fig. 8.2. Correlation in insulin-treated diabetic patients between B-cell function as measured by plasma C-peptide concentration and glycaemic control (measured by HbA_1). Preservation of even some degree of B-cell function (e.g. in the first few years after diagnosis in IDDM) is associated with relatively good control.

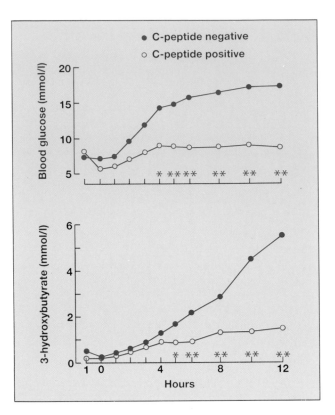

Fig. 8.3. Changes in blood glucose and 3-hydroxybutyrate concentrations in response to insulin withdrawal in IDDM patients with B-cell function (detectable C-peptide) or without B-cell function (undetectable C-peptide). C-peptide-positive patients are partially protected from metabolic decompensation. Statistical significance of differences between the two groups: $* = p < 0.05$; $**, p < 0.01$.

9: Treatment of insulin-dependent diabetes mellitus

Insulin injection therapy and blood glucose self-monitoring

● Many types of insulin injection regimen are available. Intermediate- or long-acting insulins injected once or twice daily provide the basal requirement and short-acting insulin injected 30–40 min before meals covers the additional prandial needs (Fig. 9.1).

● A common problem with twice-daily inter-mediate- and short-acting insulins is the relatively short action profile of the intermediate insulin, which when injected in the early evening tends to run out in the few hours before breakfast and so exacerbates fasting hyperglycaemia. This may be overcome by injecting the intermediate-acting insulin before bedtime (Fig. 9.2).

● The action profiles of lente and isophane in-sulins are indistinguishable in everyday use (Fig.

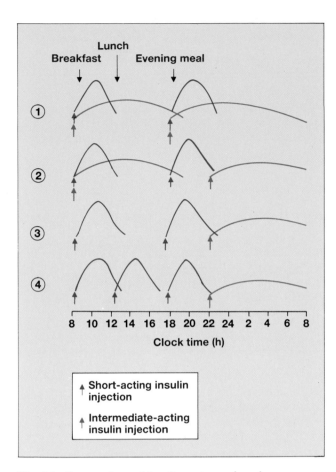

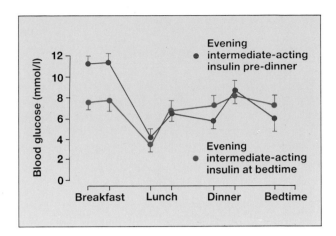

Fig. 9.2. Effect of delaying the evening injection of intermediate-acting insulin until bedtime. Mean ± SEM blood glucose values in six IDDM patients treated by twice-daily short- and intermediate-acting insulin injections. Samples were collected at home and analysed later in the laboratory. Evening intermediate-acting insulin given at bedtime reduces pre-breakfast hyperglycaemia.

Fig. 9.1. Commonly-used insulin regimens based on subcutaneous injections of short- and intermediate-acting (isophane or lente) insulins. Short-acting insulin is given before meals. Intermediate-acting insulin provides the basal insulin supply; the evening injection may be delayed until bed-time to guard against insulin deficiency before breakfast (see Fig. 9.2).

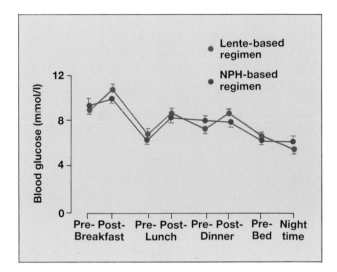

Fig. 9.3. The glycaemic equivalence of regimens based on isophane insulin or lente insulin. Mean ± SEM blood glucose values from samples collected by patients on filter paper and analysed in the laboratory.

9.3). However, excess zinc ions in lente (and ultra-lente) insulins may combine with soluble insulin when the two are mixed, significantly retarding the action profile of the short-acting component (Fig. 9.4). This problem does not occur with iso-phane insulins.

• Ultralente formulations using human insulin have a significantly shorter action profile than the original bovine preparation which was often effective when injected once daily. Human ultra-lente insulin may require two injections per day (Fig. 9.5).

• Premixed (biphasic) combinations of short-with intermediate-acting insulin may achieve good glycaemic control in patients with residual endogenous insulin secretion but are often not flexible enough for C-peptide-deficient IDDM patients.

• 'Pen devices' containing prefilled cartridges of

soluble or isophane insulin are convenient to use and popular with patients, but their use does not apparently improve glycaemic control (Fig. 9.6, Table 9.1).

• Insulin should be injected into the abdomen, outer thigh, buttock or upper arm, ideally in a fixed rotation to reduce variability in insulin absorption (Fig. 9.7). Because of the possibility of vertical injections entering muscle in thin patients, injections should probably be given at

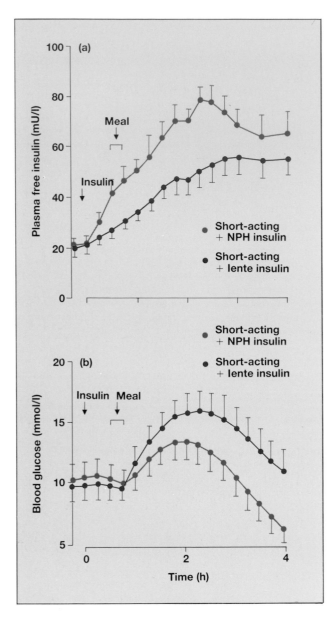

Fig. 9.4. The effect of mixing short-acting insulin with isophane or lente insulins. (a) Plasma free insulin levels after injection of isophane or lente; (b) equivalent blood glucose concentrations. Excess zinc ions in lente insulin combine with short-acting insulin on mixing, thereby reducing the rise in plasma-free insulin and increasing post-prandial hyperglycaemia.

an angle into a pinched-up skin fold. There is no need to clean the skin.

• Disposable syringes can safely be re-used for at least 7 days, and needles until they become blunt. Infections at insulin injection sites are very rare.

• Some benefits of blood glucose self-monitoring are outlined in Table 9.2, and some of the reasons why problems may be encountered are listed in Table 9.3.

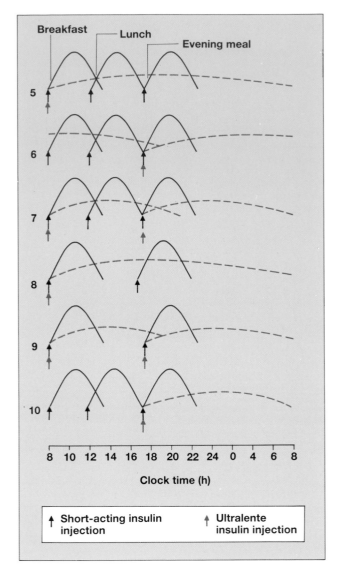

Fig. 9.5. Commonly used insulin regimens based on subcutaneous injections of short-acting and ultralente-type insulins. Ultralente insulin provides the basal insulin supply and may be given once or twice a day.

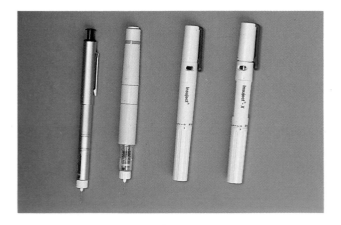

Fig. 9.6. Insulin 'pens' (left to right: NovoPen I, NovoPen II, Insuject, Insuject X; Novo–Nordisk).

Table 9.1. Advantages of insulin 'pens'.

- *Convenience* — not necessary to carry syringe, needle and insulin vial
- *Patient acceptance* — encourages use of multiple insulin injection regimens; injections less painful
- *Speed* — quicker than conventional injection techniques
- *Ease* — possible to inject with one-handed technique

Table 9.2. Some benefits of blood glucose self-monitoring.

More accurate and patient-acceptable than urine tests for glucose

Provides information for feedback control of insulin delivery
- on a day-to-day basis, by the patient
- in the long-term, by the physician

Defines the level of glycaemic control achieved
- for research
- for routine clinical assessment

Identifies hypoglycaemia
- impossible with urine testing
- particularly valuable in patients with loss of hypoglycaemic awareness

Acts as an educational aid

Increases patient participation, motivation and interest

Reinforces the patient's feeling of being 'in control', thus offering independence, shared responsibility and self-confidence.

Improves quality of life

Allows the patient to relate level of control to feeling of well-being

Reduces hospital admission (?)

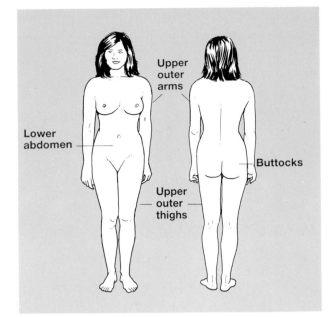

Fig. 9.7. Suitable sites for subcutaneous insulin injection. Injections should be rotated within a given area to reduce lipohypertrophy. Injection is probably best given into a lifted skin fold to avoid inadvertent intramuscular injection.

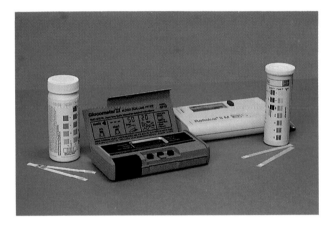

Fig. 9.8. Glucose oxidase reagent strips and reflectance meters (left to right: Glucostix and Glucometer II (Ames); Reflolux II and BM Test 1–44 Strips (Boehringer Mannheim).

- Reagent strips for blood glucose measurement contain glucose oxidase immobilized together with peroxidase and a chromogen whose colour changes on exposure to the hydrogen peroxide generated by glucose oxidation (Fig. 9.8).
- Reagent strips can be compared visually against a standard colour chart, or read using a reflectance meter. Meters are useful for patients with colour vision defects due to retinopathy or other causes.
- Blood for glucose monitoring should be obtained by pricking the sides of the fingertips, rather than the sensitive pulps. The blood drop must be applied correctly to the strip and the reaction timed precisely in order to achieve accurate results (Fig. 9.9).

Table 9.3. Some reasons for poor results with blood glucose self-monitoring (BGSM).

Poor training in technique of BGSM
Reflectance meter fault
Poor eyesight (e.g. because of age, retinopathy, colour-vision defects)
Poor timing of tests
Insufficiently large blood sample
Incorrect removal of blood sample from strip
Out-of-date or improperly stored test strips
Altered haematocrit
Overt misinterpretation of readings
Deliberate mis-recording of results (e.g. omission of very high and low results)

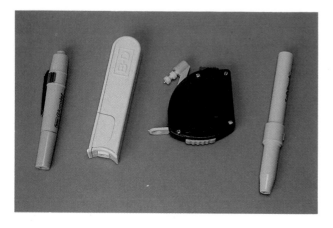

Fig. 9.9. Devices for automatic finger pricking (left to right): Glucolet (Ames), Autolance (Becton-Dickinson), Autolet II (Owen Mumford), and Soft Touch (Boehringer Mannheim).

● Algorithms (sequences of rules) for adjusting insulin dosages and food intake according to blood glucose values can be drawn up for individual patients (Table 9.4).

● Patients who are not acutely ill (i.e. vomiting) may begin insulin treatment outside hospital if under the close supervision of a diabetes specialist nurse. Initial insulin dosages should be low (e.g. 6–10 units of intermediate-acting insulin twice-daily) to avoid hypoglycaemia (Table 9.5).

Diet

● The nutritional requirements of people with IDDM are similar to those of non-diabetic subjects (Table 9.6). Dietary management in IDDM should aim in the short-term to prevent hypoglycaemia and in the long-term to reduce the risks of chronic diabetic complications.

● Fat should provide ≤30% of total energy for a person with IDDM. *Saturated* fat should account for ≤10%, the remainder comprising monounsaturated fats (e.g. olive oil) and polyunsaturated fats (e.g. other vegetable and fish oils) which may improve the lipaemic profile, reducing LDL cholesterol and increasing HDL cholesterol levels. Fat intake up to 35% of energy is acceptable when the extra comes mainly from monounsaturated fats, e.g. olive oil in Mediterranean diets.

● Carbohydrate should provide >55% of total energy intake. Complex carbohydrates (starch-rich foods) should predominate but moderate amounts of simple sugars (up to 25 g per day) are probably acceptable. High-carbohydrate diets only improve blood glucose and lipid levels if accompanied by at least 30 g/day of dietary fibre, particularly the 'soluble fibre', found in vegetables, pulses, fruits and whole grain cereals; this is nearly twice as high as the average British intake.

● Protein should contribute about 10–15% to total energy intake with emphasis on vegetable sources. High-protein diets may accelerate the progression of diabetic nephropathy.

● Dietary recommendations must be carefully adapted to each patient's individual needs; children and people from ethnic minorities require special consideration.

● Food exchange systems help to keep the diet

Table 9.4. Simple algorithm for adjusting insulin dosage by BGSM, for patients receiving twice-daily short- and intermediate-acting insulins.

● *Target blood glucose levels:*
Before meals: 4–6 mmol/l
After meals: less than 10 mmol/l

● *If blood glucose result is too high for 2 days or more:*

Before breakfast	Before lunch	Before evening meal	At bedtime
Increase evening long-acting insulin	Increase morning short-acting insulin	Increase morning long-acting insulin	Increase evening short-acting insulin

● *If blood glucose result is too low for 2 days or more:*

Before breakfast	Before lunch	Before evening meal	At bedtime
Reduce evening long-acting insulin	Reduce morning short-acting insulin	Reduce morning long-acting insulin	Reduce evening short-acting insulin

Note: Increase or decrease insulin by 2 U at a time.

Table 9.5. Programme for starting insulin treatment as an outpatient.

1st session
Short talk with physician (~ 30 min)
One-to-one instruction by diabetes nurse specialist
Nurse demonstrates drawing up of insulin dose and injection technique
Patient injects himself with insulin
Patient learns to draw up insulin
Starting insulin dosage: 6−10 U intermediate-acting insulin twice-daily
'Survival' information
 • recognition and treatment of hypoglycaemia
 • reassurance about specific anxieties
 • advice on driving and work
 • contact telephone number of nurse and doctor
 • advice to eat regular meals (no specific diet instruction)

After 1 week
Review above

After 2 weeks
Teach BGSM
Full dietary instruction

varied while maintaining the daily pattern of food intake. Exchanges based on whole meals may be preferable to those concentrating on the carbohydrate content of different foods.
• Sodium intake should not exceed 6 g/day; a reduction to ≤3 g/day may reduce blood pressure.
• Alcohol intake, as in the general population, should not exceed 3 units per day in men, and 2 U/day in women. 'Diabetic' beverages have low sugar but high alcohol contents, increasing the risks of hypoglycaemia, and should therefore be avoided.
• 'Diabetic' foods and sweets are often expensive, unpalatable, and associated with gastrointestinal side-effects. They have no nutritional or metabolic benefits and should be avoided. Low-energy sweeteners such as saccharine or aspartame are safe and useful in obese patients.
• Regular daily exercise (20 min of moderate exertion) is recommended for diabetic as for non-diabetic people. Hypoglycaemia during or after exercise can be minimized by carefully timing exercise and eating, by reducing pre-exercise insulin dosages and by taking 'slow-release' carbohydrate in foods before exertion.

Continuous subcutaneous insulin infusion (CSII)

• Continuous subcutaneous insulin infusion (CSII) mimics non-diabetic insulin delivery by infusing insulin from a portable pump at an adjustable basal rate with patient-activated boosts before meals (Figs 9.10, 9.11).
• The infusion strategy used for starting patients on CSII is outlined in Fig. 9.12. Patients started on CSII must receive comprehensive education, including details of pump operation, home blood

Table 9.6. General principles of diet for diabetic patients, as compared with the current average diet in Britain.

	Recommendations for diabetes mellitus	Approximate content of usual UK diet
Energy intake	To approach BMI 22	Maintains BMI 24−25
Carbohydrate	>55% of energy	45% of energy
Fat	<30−35% of energy* (saturated fat <10%)	42% of energy
Protein	10−15% of energy	12% of energy
Salt	<6 g daily (<3 g if hypertensive)	10 g daily
Sucrose (added)	<25 g daily	50−100 g daily
Dietary fibre	>30 g daily	20 g daily
Special so-called 'diabetic' foods	None (avoid)	None

BMI: body mass index (weight in kg/(height in m)^2.
* A higher total fat content is permissible when monounsaturated fatty acids form a major component, as from olive oil in Mediterranean diets.

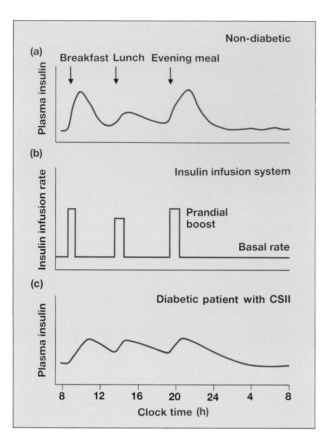

Fig. 9.10. The simulation of non-diabetic insulin secretory profiles by open-loop insulin infusion, e.g. CSII; (a) plasma insulin levels in a non-diabetic subject; (b) basal infusion and prandial boost of CSII mimicking non-diabetic insulin secretion; (c) resultant plasma free insulin levels in diabetic subjects treated by CSII.

glucose monitoring, insulin dosage adjustments and corrective action in case of illness, hypoglycaemia, hyperglycaemia or pump breakdown (Table 9.7).

• CSII should only be undertaken by centres which can provide supervision by experienced staff and a 24-h telephone service for immediate advice about management problems (Table 9.8).

• Long-term strict control of blood glucose, intermediary metabolites and hormones can be obtained with CSII (Fig. 9.13), although (as with insulin injection treatment) at the expense of higher blood insulin levels than in non-diabetic subjects.

• CSII is an alternative form of intensified insulin therapy for IDDM patients and may be used for experimental studies, e.g. investigating the links between control and diabetic complications. Routine treatment by CSII is suitable for a relatively small number of selected patients.

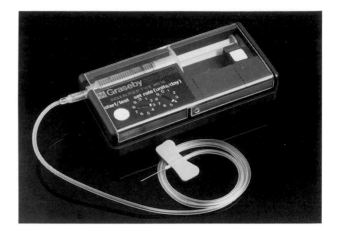

Fig. 9.11. An insulin infusion pump used for CSII.

Table 9.7. Education and information about CSII.

• Explain the principles of CSII, why CSII is being undertaken, how to operate the pump and what to do in emergencies (see below) to both the patient and relatives or partners who will be with the patient at home.
• Demonstrate the pump and how it works, the alarms, battery insertion and expected lifetime, adjustment of basal rate, activation of mealtime boost, cannula insertion and its securing to skin, and cannula changes.
• Re-educate about blood glucose self-monitoring and urinary ketone monitoring and teach simple rules for basal and preprandial dosage adjustments.
• Provide general and CSII-related dieting advice, noting possible weight gain but opportunities for more flexibility at mealtimes.
• Give instructions on CSII and exercise, sports, bathing and sexual intercourse.
• Give instructions for action in case of hypo- and hyperglycaemia, intercurrent illness, ketonuria, infusion site problems and pump breakdown.
• Give information about 24-h on-call telephone service for contacting hospital.
• Supply insulin and syringes for emergency reversion to injection therapy.
• Supply with identification card (e.g. 'I am a diabetic receiving insulin via an infusion pump. In the event of an emergency please telephone Dr X at Y Hospital').

Table 9.8. When to consider CSII.

• When optimized conventional insulin injection treatment has failed (e.g. in some hypoglycaemia-prone diabetic subjects)
• When the centre has special expertise and experience of CSII
• When the patient prefers CSII (e.g. dislikes multiple injections)
• When the patient has an erratic lifestyle (more flexibility to omit or delay mealtimes).

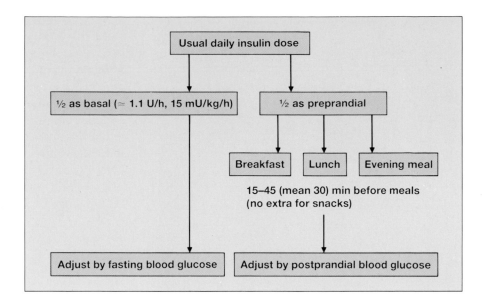

Fig. 9.12. The infusion strategy used for starting patients on CSII.

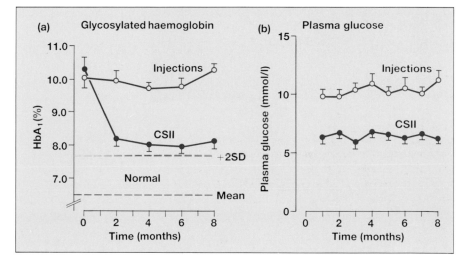

Fig. 9.13. Glycaemic control in patients randomly assigned to continued conventional insulin injection therapy (○) or CSII (●); (a) changes in glycosylated haemoglobin (HbA₁); (b) changes in plasma glucose levels calculated from home-collected samples taken throughout the day (mean ± SEM).

Anti-insulin antibodies: a complication of insulin therapy

- Insulin, together with its polymers and other chemical derivatives, is immunogenic. Bovine insulin is more immunogenic than porcine; human-sequence insulin is the least immunogenic but can none the less provoke antibody formation. Highly purified insulins have low immunogenicity.
- Insulin-binding antibodies (mostly polyclonal) are detectable in most insulin-treated patients but in most cases are clinically irrelevant.
- The binding of insulin to antibody is governed by the law of mass action; only free (or unbound) insulin is thought to be biologically active.

- Insulin antibodies may 'buffer' against sudden fluctuations in free insulin levels under experimental conditions, but generally do not seem to influence clinical insulin requirements or metabolic stability.
- The clinical manifestations of insulin antibodies, now rare, include:
1 local allergic reactions (either immediate, IgE-mediated, or delayed Arthus-type reactions due to IgG immune complexes) and possibly lipoatrophy at injection sites (Fig. 9.14);
2 anaphylaxis, due to IgE antibody formation; and insulin resistance, due to rapid clearance of injected insulin which forms large immune complexes with polyclonal antibodies.
- Treatment of these problems is by substituting

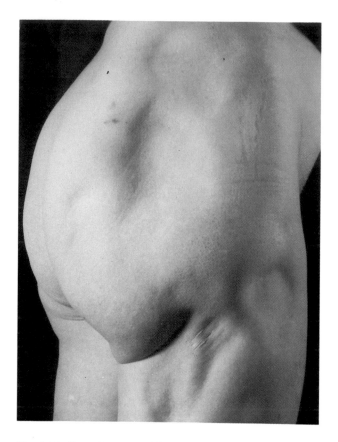

Fig. 9.14. Extensive areas of lipoatrophy in a 39-year-old woman treated for over 20 years with various 'impure' insulin preparations, including protamine-zinc.

another insulin species which does not cross-react with the antibodies, by desensitization, or by local or systemic administration of glucocorticoids.

● Insulin autoantibodies can develop without previous exposure to exogenous insulin in some patients receiving methimazole or other drugs, and may cause a syndrome of postprandial glucose intolerance combined with fasting hypoglycaemia.

● Insulin autoantibodies also occur in 30–40% of IDDM children at presentation and in their high-risk siblings, and may be a marker for the 'prediabetic' stage of IDDM.

10: Treatment of non-insulin-dependent diabetes mellitus

Diet

● The energy-dense 'Westernized' diet, rich in fats and relatively low in carbohydrate and fibre, is a major cause of obesity and a contributor to NIDDM. Dietary modification, concentrating on fat restriction, to reduce energy intake and body weight, should be the starting point and mainstay of long-term treatment of NIDDM.

● Reducing energy intake acutely reduces glycaemia and diabetic symptoms (Fig. 10.1), even before significant weight loss occurs, but achieving full glycaemic and metabolic normalization may require considerable weight loss (Table 10.1).

● Weight loss reduces cardiovascular risk factors, lowering blood pressure and the atherogenicity of blood lipid profiles, and extends the life expectancy of NIDDM patients (Table 10.2).

● The current energy intake of an individual patient, the necessary energy restriction for slimming and the expected rate of weight loss during a given diet, are all best estimated from standard formulae (Table 10.3); trying to use dietary records is unreliable, because overweight patients greatly underestimate their food intake.

● Simple initial advice (Table 10.4) must be followed by a full dietary assessment and prescription of an appropriate regimen.

● Changing to a high-carbohydrate, high-fibre,

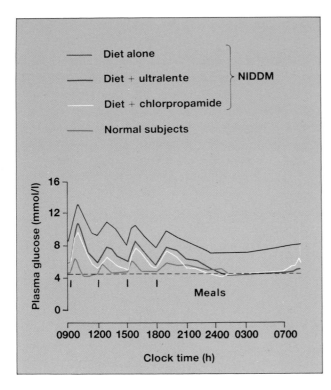

Legend:
— Diet alone
— Diet + ultralente — NIDDM
— Diet + chlorpropamide
— Normal subjects

Fig. 10.1. Twenty four-hour plasma glucose concentrations in a group of NIDDM patients treated initially by diet alone and then by diet with chlorpropamide or ultralente insulin in sufficient doses to reduce the basal plasma glucose concentration to 6 mmol/l. Postprandial glycaemic excursions remain large but overall glycaemic exposure is considerably reduced. Note how the fasting plasma glucose concentration is a good indicator of overall glycaemic control throughout the day during each of the different therapies.

Table 10.1. Benefits of reduced energy intake and weight loss in NIDDM.

Acute energy restriction before detectable weight loss
Marked fall in blood glucose concentrations
Symptomatic improvement

Long-term energy restriction, with significant weight loss
Gradual fall (possibly normalization) of blood glucose concentrations
Improved insulin sensitivity
Reduced atherogenicity of blood lipid profiles
Fall in blood pressure
Increased life expectancy

Table 10.2. Advantages of high-carbohydrate, low-fat diets for slimming and maintenance of weight loss in NIDDM subjects.

Lower energy density of carbohydrate ⎫ Increased bulk,
Higher dietary fibre content ⎬ more satisfying
Improved insulin sensitivity ⎭
Reduced hyperinsulinaemia (? reduced GIP-mediated stimulation of insulin secretion)
Increased diet-induced thermogenesis, therefore increased energy expenditure
If overeaten, less tendency to fat deposition (energy expended in converting carbohydrate into fatty acids for storage)

low-fat diet sometimes increases body water and weight initially, but will often lead to weight loss even without overall energy restriction. Such diets stimulate energy expenditure, reduce hyperinsulinaemia and the tendency to fat deposition, and improve atherogenic lipaemic profiles.

● Most NIDDM patients cannot comply with

Table 10.3. Predicting weight loss during different diets in subjects aged 30–60 years. Note that the expected weight loss during a fixed energy intake (e.g. 1000 kcal/day) increases with increasing body weight. This is because — contrary to popular belief — obese people expend more energy than the non-obese.

Weight (kg)		Mean (range) weight loss (kg/month)		
		1000 kcal/day	1500 kcal/day	2000 kcal/day
70–80	Male	5.0 (3.1–6.8)	2.8 (1.0–4.7)	0.7 (0–2.5)
	Female	3.5 (1.9–5.0)	1.4 (0–2.9)	0 (0–0.7)
80–90	Male	5.6 (3.6–7.6)	3.4 (1.5–5.4)	1.3 (0–3.3)
	Female	3.9 (2.3–5.6)	1.8 (0.2–3.5)	0 (0–1.3)
90–100	Male	6.2 (4.1–8.2)	4.1 (2.0–6.1)	2.0 (0–4.0)
	Female	4.4 (2.6–6.1)	2.3 (0.5–4.0)	0.2 (0–1.8)
100–110	Male	6.8 (4.6–9.0)	4.7 (2.5–6.9)	2.6 (0.4–4.9)
	Female	4.8 (3.0–6.6)	2.7 (0.9–4.5)	0.6 (0–2.3)
110–120	Male	7.4 (5.1–9.8)	5.3 (3.2–7.7)	3.2 (0.8–5.5)
	Female	5.2 (3.3–7.1)	3.1 (2.2–5.0)	0.9 (0–2.8)

These predictions assume that total daily energy expenditure = 1.25 × BMR and that expenditure will be suppressed by 15% following weight loss. The ranges are calculated for BMR ±20% of average.
Notes: **1** Initial weight loss will be more rapid; **2** Regular exercise will accelerate weight loss; **3** Subjects aged over 60 years will lose weight more slowly: subtract 1.4 kg/month for men and 0.6 kg/month for women.

slimming diets and fail to reach their ideal weight. Dietary advice must take account of individual dietary preferences, attitudes and life-style as well as the degree of overweight. A 'target' weight and the time taken to achieve it should be based on realistic predictions of weight loss. These can be calculated from Table 10.3.

• Slimming diets should aim for an energy deficit of 500 kcal/day, leading to weight loss of about 0.5 kg/week. Weight loss should not exceed 2–3 kg/week, as this suggests excessive loss of muscle rather than fat.

• Diets containing less than 700 kcal/day (very low calorie diets) with adequate vitamin and mineral supplements have not been shown to produce better long-term results than conventional slimming diets and may be contraindicated in NIDDM because of the uncertain risks of subclinical heart disease.

• Dietary supplementation with soluble fibre can improve glycaemic and lipaemic profiles in NIDDM. Fish oil and vegetable preparations rich in essential fatty acids also improve blood lipids but the former may worsen hyperglycaemia in NIDDM patients.

• Regular exercise taken in conjunction with energy restriction will enhance weight loss in NIDDM patients and maximize loss of fat while preserving muscle. Advice regarding exercise must be appropriate to the patient's lifestyle, physical condition and capability.

Table 10.4. Initial dietary advice for a newly diagnosed diabetic patient (IDDM or NIDDM).

• Drink *water* to quench thirst
• Eat to appetite with *normal foods*; take regular meals
• Make the *main part of each meal* cereal, bread or pasta
• Make meat or cheese a *small* part of each meal

Oral agents and insulin

• Patients with NIDDM characteristically have an elevated basal blood glucose level on which is superimposed exaggerated postprandial glycaemic excursions (Fig. 10.1).

• The fasting blood glucose (FBG) level provides a single, reproducible and reliable indicator of overall glycaemic control and, in practice, it is this basal hyperglycaemia which responds most easily to treatment (Fig. 10.1).

• The primary therapy in NIDDM remains adjustment of dietary content and, if feasible, increased exercise. In practice, only 15% of patients can achieve fasting plasma glucose values below 6 mmol/l by dietary manipulation alone and of these less than one-half can maintain fasting normoglycaemia for more than 1 year.

• In these cases oral agents may be given. Table 10.5 describes the pharmacokinetic and prescribing information for a range of sulphonylureas. First and second generation drugs are generally comparable, but the long-acting chlorpropamide and the potent glibenclamide are best avoided in the elderly because of the increased risk of hypoglycaemia.

• After diet therapy has been tried, oral agents only achieve an FBG<6 mmol/l in approximately 50% of patients. Strategies for treating patients who fail to respond to diet alone depend on whether the aim is to try and normalize glycaemia (Table 10.6) or alleviate symptoms (Table 10.7).

• 'Sulphonylurea failure' is an outdated term which describes persistence or recurrence of glycosuric symptoms during treatment. This depends on both glycaemia and the renal threshold. *Primary failure*, with continued symptoms despite sulphonylurea therapy, is likely when FBG exceeds

Table 10.5. Sulphonylureas: pharmacokinetic and prescribing information. The year in which each drug was introduced is shown in parentheses.

First generation	Dose range	Dose distribution	Half-life
Tolbutamide (1956)	1.0–3.0 g	Divided	3–8 h
Chlorpropamide (1957)	100–500 mg	Single daily	35 h
Acetohexamide (1962)	0.25–1.5 g	Single or divided	6–8 h
Tolazamide (1962)	100–750 mg	Single or divided	7 h
Second generation			
Glymidine (1964)	0.5–2.0 g	Single or divided	4 h
Glibenclamide (1969)	2.5–20 mg	Single or divided	5 h
Glibornuride (1970)	12.5–75 mg	Single or divided	8 h
Glipizide (1971)	2.5–20 mg	Single or divided	4 h
Gliclazide (1979)	80–320 mg	Single or divided	12 h
Gliquidone (1975)	60–180 mg	Single or divided	4 h

Table 10.6. Guide to therapy in NIDDM when aiming for basal normoglycaemia (FBG < 6 mmol/l).

Current therapy	Fasting blood glucose (mmol/l)	Suggested action
Diet only	6–8	Add chlorpropamide 100 mg/day
	8–10	Add chlorpropamide 250 mg/day
	10–12	Add chlorpropamide 500 mg/day
	12–18	Add chlorpropamide 500 mg/day but will almost certainly require an additional therapeutic agent
	> 18	Add basal and prandial insulin
Maximum chlorpropamide	6–8	Add metformin 500 mg twice daily
	8–12	Add once-daily ultralente insulin
	>12	Stop chlorpropamide. Start basal and prandial insulin
Maximum chlorpropamide + maximum metformin	6–10	Stop metformin Add once-daily ultralente insulin Stop chlorpropamide and metformin
	>10	Start basal and prandial insulin
Maximum chlorpropamide + ultralente insulin	Preprandial blood glucose >7	Stop chlorpropamide Add prandial insulin

Note: Chlorpropamide is shown as an example. Other sulphonylureas may be substituted.

Table 10.7. Guide to therapy in NIDDM when aiming to abolish symptoms and to reduce the fasting blood glucose to below 10 mmol/l.

Current therapy	Fasting-blood glucose (mmol/l)	Suggested action
Diet only	6–8	Add chlorpropamide 100 mg/day
	8–10	Add chlorpropamide 250 mg/day
	10–18	Add chlorpropamide 500 mg/day
	18–25	Add chlorpropamide 500 mg/day but will almost certainly require an additional therapeutic agent
	>25	Add once-daily insulin, e.g. lente ± soluble mixture
Maximum chlorpropamide	6–10	Continue maximum chlorpropamide
	10–14	Add metformin 500 mg twice daily
	14–20	Add once-daily ultralente insulin
	>20	Stop chlorpropamide. Start once-daily insulin, e.g. lente ± soluble mixture
Maximum chlorpropamide + maximum metformin	6–10	Continue maximum chlorpropamide and metformin
	10–20	Stop metformin Add once-daily ultralente insulin
	>20	Stop chlorpropamide and metformin Start once-daily insulin, e.g. lente ± soluble mixture
Maximum chlorpropamide + ultralente insulin	>20 or symptoms	Stop chlorpropamide and ultralente Start insulin, e.g. once-daily lente ± soluble insulin or twice-daily soluble isophane

14 mmol/l and occurs in about 5% of patients. *Secondary* failure, with symptoms recurring months or years after initial therapeutic success, is probably due to progressively deteriorating B-cell function. An additional term, sulphonylurea inadequacy, describes patients who continue to

Table 10.8. Guide to doses required in NIDDM for a basal insulin supplement to diet and oral agents for an average 5' 10" (1.78 m) person. Dosages are suggested according to the fasting blood glucose level and degree of obesity. It is assumed that the patient will maintain the same diet and oral therapy and remains in good health. The doses are those suitable for starting as an outpatient and will need to be altered according to the glycaemic control achieved. Patients should be warned about the possibility of hypoglycaemia although this is rarely a problem with these doses. Most patients will eventually need 20–30% more than these doses to obtain a fasting blood glucose below 6 mmol/l.

	Fasting blood glucose (mmol/l)	Patients with ideal body weight	% over ideal body weight				
			+20	+40	+60	+80	+100
Males	6	6	9	12	15	18	21
	8	10	15	20	25	30	35
	10	14	21	28	35	42	49
	12	18	27	36	45	54	63
	>14	22	33	44	55	66	77
Females	6	5	7	9	11	14	16
	8	8	11	15	19	23	26
	10	11	16	21	26	32	37
	12	14	20	27	34	41	47
	>14	17	25	33	41	50	58

have an FBG > 6 mmol/l despite maximal sulphonylurea therapy.

• When near-normal FBG levels cannot be achieved with a combination of sulphonylurea and metformin, improved glycaemic control can often be achieved by a long-acting insulin preparation, such as ultralente (Tables 10.6 & 10.7). The advantages of combined insulin and sulphonylurea therapy over a basal insulin supplement alone are that less exogenous insulin is needed and slightly better glucose control may be obtained with the enhanced endogenous insulin secretion, particularly when insulin resistance is increased, as with intercurrent infections.

• For combined insulin and sulphonylurea therapy, insulin dosages are suggested according to the fasting blood glucose level, and the degree of obesity (Table 10.8).

• Full insulin treatment, with prandial as well as basal injections, is needed in more severely insulin-deficient patients with persistent post-prandial hyperglycaemia (Table 10.9). A guide to prandial insulin doses in NIDDM is given in Table 10.10. Sulphonylurea therapy is of little benefit in these patients and should be stopped. Careful glycaemic monitoring and attention to diet and exercise are then needed.

Table 10.10. Guide to prandial insulin doses in NIDDM. This table assumes that the patient is receiving a basal dose which maintains the fasting blood glucose at 4–6 mmol/l. Determine the patient's percentage of ideal body weight and read off the prandial dose which corresponds to the empirical basal requirement.

This is the *total* daily prandial requirement and will need to be subdivided according to meal-size and exercise. Final adjustments must be on the basis of glycaemic monitoring.

	Ideal weight	% over ideal body weight				
		+20	+40	+60	+80	+100
Basal	16	24	32	40	48	56
Prandial	2	3	4	5	6	7
Basal	20	30	40	50	60	70
Prandial	6	9	12	15	18	21
Basal	24	36	48	60	72	84
Prandial	10	15	20	25	30	35
Basal	28	42	56	70	84	98
Prandial	18	27	36	45	54	63
Basal	32	48	64	80	96	112
Prandial	28	42	56	70	84	98
Basal	36	54	72	90	108	126
Prandial	42	63	84	105	126	147

Table 10.9. Features suggesting the need for full (basal and prandial) insulin treatment in NIDDM patients.

• FBG with diet alone >12 mmol/l
• FBG with diet plus maximal oral agents >10 mmol/l
• Blood glucose remains >7 mmol/l before meals when treated with ultralente alone
• Raised HbA$_{1c}$ but normal FBG when treated with ultralente alone
• Basal insulin requirement >14 U/day in lean patients (>0.2 U/kg/day in obese)

11: Hypoglycaemia and diabetes

• Over 30% of insulin-treated diabetic patients experience hypoglycaemic coma at least once, about 10% suffer coma in any one year, and about 3% are incapacitated by frequent and severe episodes.

• Hypoglycaemia kills at least 3−4% of insulin-treated diabetic patients. Glycaemic thresholds for the onset of symptoms as acute hypoglycaemia develops in non-diabetic subjects are shown in Fig. 11.1.

• Hypoglycaemia in diabetic patients is often due to mismatching of hypoglycaemic medication, food and exercise.

• Intensification of insulin treatment alone need not in itself cause more frequent or severe hypoglycaemia, but may blunt symptomatic awareness of it.

• Reduced insulin requirements during the 'honeymoon period', after delivery, or following weight loss or the onset of adrenal or pituitary failure, may predispose to hypoglycaemia.

• Mild neuroglycopenia (blood glucose concentration ≤3.0 mmol/l) produces subtle intellectual and psychomotor impairment; severe neuroglycopenia (blood glucose ≤1.0 mmol/l) causes confusion, disturbed behaviour, fits and ultimately unconsciousness. Permanent brain damage is unusual after hypoglycaemic coma, but more likely in people with excessive alcohol intake.

• Generalized autonomic activation (triggered by blood glucose ≤2.0 mmol/l) causes tremor, tachycardia, sweating, altered salivation and hunger.

• Awareness of hypoglycaemia may be reduced or lost in IDDM patients, especially those with long-standing disease; autonomic neuropathy or the effect of intensified insulin treatment may be partly responsible.

• Reduced hypoglycaemia awareness in a few patients following transfer from animal to human insulin is probably due, in most cases, to altered regimens and improved glycaemic control.

• Recovery from hypoglycaemia depends on glucose counter-regulation, mediated largely by hormones opposing insulin's action, namely glucagon, adrenaline, growth hormone, cortisol and vasopressin (Fig. 11.2). Recovery may be delayed by deficiencies of these counter-regulatory hormones (common in long-standing IDDM) and by

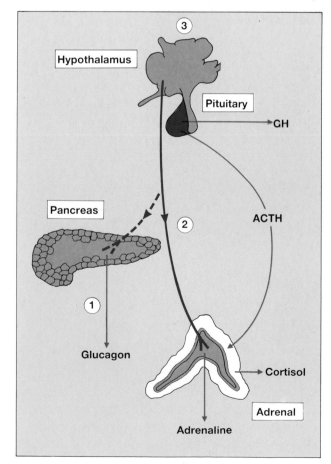

Fig. 11.2 Principal counter-regulatory mechanisms in humans, releasing glucagon, adrenaline, cortisol and growth hormone (GH). In diabetes, deficiencies can occur at different sites: (1) intrinsic pancreatic A-cell secretion; (2) autonomic neuropathy; (3) diminished central activation of glucose counter-regulation.

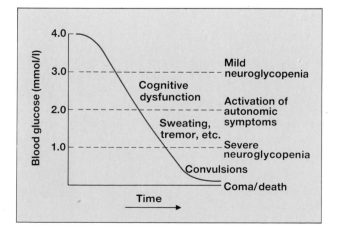

Fig. 11.1. Glycaemic thresholds for onset of symptoms of acute hypoglycaemia in non-diabetic subjects.

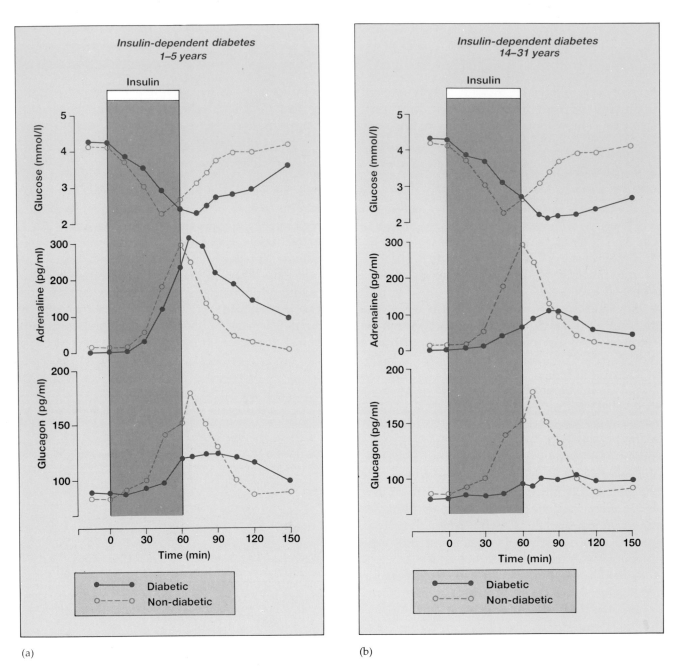

(a)

(b)

Fig. 11.3. The effect of diabetes duration on recovery from insulin-induced hypoglycaemia and its relationship to counter-regulatory hormone release. (a) With IDDM of short duration, recovery from hypoglycaemia is delayed compared to the non-diabetic person. The main defect is a reduced release of glucagon in response to hypoglycaemia. Catecholamine responses remain essentially unaltered. (b) With IDDM of long duration, glycaemic recovery is severely impaired due to deficiencies in both glucagon and catecholamine release after hypoglycaemia.

non-selective β-adrenergic blockade (Fig. 11.3).

● Sulphonylurea-induced hypoglycaemia affects about 20 in 1000 patients per year; it is more common with long-acting agents such as chlorpropamide and glibenclamide, which should therefore be avoided in the elderly.

● Glycaemic control may have to be relaxed in patients at high risk of hypoglycaemia.

● First-aid treatment of hypoglycaemia in con-scious patients is by oral administration of 15–20 g glucose. Unconscious patients should be given intravenous glucose (e.g. 30 ml of 20% solution) or glucagon (1 mg subcutaneously or intra-muscularly); there are now doubts about the efficacy of glucose gel or jam smeared inside the cheeks. Hypoglycaemia due to long-acting sul-phonylureas may require prolonged intravenous glucose infusion.

12: Diabetic ketoacidosis, non-ketotic hyperosmolar coma and lactic acidosis

- Coma or impaired consciousness in diabetic patients may have several causes, including diabetic ketoacidosis, diabetic non-ketotic hyperosmolar coma, and lactic acidosis (Table 12.1).

Diabetic ketoacidosis

- Diabetic ketoacidosis is the largest single cause of death in diabetic patients under the age of 20 years in the UK, with an average mortality of about 7% of episodes. Mortality is particularly high in the elderly.
- The common precipitating causes are infection, management errors and new cases of diabetes, but there is no obvious cause in about 40% of episodes (Fig. 12.1). The main causes of death are shown in Table 12.2.
- Ketoacidosis is initiated by an absolute or relative insulin deficiency and an increase in catabolic hormones, leading to hepatic over-production of glucose and ketone bodies.
- Symptoms include increasing polyuria and polydipsia, weight loss, weakness, drowsiness and eventual coma (10% of cases); abdominal pain may be present, particularly in the young (Table 12.3).
- Signs include dehydration, hypotension, tachycardia, hyperventilation and hypothermia.
- Immediate investigations should include bedside blood glucose and ketone estimations by reagent strips, followed by laboratory measurements of blood glucose, urea, Na^+, K^+, full blood count, arterial blood pH (and gases in shocked patients), and blood and urine culture in all subjects.

Table 12.1. Causes of coma or impaired consciousness in diabetic patients.

- Diabetic ketoacidosis
- Hyperosmolar, hyperglycaemic, non-ketotic coma
- Hypoglycaemia
- Lactic acidosis
- Other causes (sometimes related to diabetes):
  stroke
  postictal (including hypoglycaemia)
  trauma
  drug overdose, ethanol intoxication

Table 12.2. Principal causes of mortality occurring in 746 episodes of diabetic ketoacidosis.

Cause of death	Number of deaths
Primary metabolic causes	10
Myocardial infarction/ congestive cardiac failure	9
Pneumonia	7
Pulmonary emboli	3
Other conditions	3
Total	32

Table 12.3. Clinical features of diabetic ketoacidosis.

Polyuria, nocturia; thirst
Weight loss
Weakness
Visual disturbance
Abdominal pain
Leg cramps
Nausea, vomiting
Confusion, drowsiness, coma

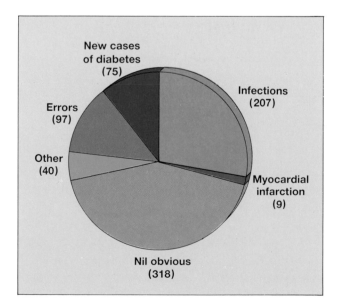

Fig. 12.1. Precipitating causes of 746 episodes of diabetic ketoacidosis observed in Birmingham, UK, during the period 1971–85.

- Table 12.4 outlines the potential pitfalls in diagnosing and managing diabetic ketoacidosis.
- Treatment involves (Table 12.5):

rehydration with isotonic saline (e.g. 2 l/h in the first 4 h, 4−6 l in the first 24 h) — shocked patients will need more rehydration while the elderly or those in cardiac failure should be rehydrated slowly and with caution.

short-acting insulin, ideally by low-dose intravenous infusion (e.g. 5−10 U/h until blood glucose level reaches 14 mmol/l, then 2−4 U/h), or by intramuscular injection (e.g. 20 U i.m. followed by 5−10 U/h until blood glucose reaches 14 mmol/l); *potassium replacement* (generally 20 mmol K^+/l of saline, adjusted by careful monitoring).

- Small doses of sodium bicarbonate (100 mmol, given as isotonic (1.4%) solution) may be given if the blood pH is <7.0 or cardiorespiratory collapse seems imminent.
- Complications of ketoacidosis include cerebral oedema (especially in the young), adult respiratory distress syndrome and thromboembolism.

- *Smell of 'ketones' (acetone) on the breath*: may be absent (many people are anosmic for acetone)
- *Fever*: may be absent (peripheral vasodilation causes cooling)
- *Leukocytosis*: neutrophil count may be non-specifically raised
- *Plasma sodium concentration*: may be artificially lowered initially by high lipid and glucose levels and may appear to rise suddenly after insulin treatment lowers plasma glucose and lipid levels
- *Plasma potassium concentration*: may be temporarily raised (by acidosis) despite severe total body potassium depletion
- *Plasma creatinine concentration*: may be falsely elevated (assay interference)
- *'Ketostix' testing*: may show negative or trace result when diabetic ketoacidosis and either lactic acidosis or alcoholic ketoacidosis coexist (predominance of 3-hydroxybutyrate).

Table 12.4. Potential pitfalls in the diagnosis and management of diabetic ketoacidosis.

Table 12.5. Initial treatment plan for diabetic ketoacidosis in adults.

Fluids and electrolytes
Volumes
- 2 l in 4 h, then 1 l in 4 h; 4−6 l in first 24 h.

Fluids
- Isotonic ('normal') saline (150 mmol/l) generally used
- Hypotonic ('half-normal') saline (75 mmol/l) if plasma sodium exceeds 150 mmol/l (1 l)
- Change to 5% glucose when blood glucose falls below 14 mmol/l
- Sodium bicarbonate (600 ml of 1.4%) if pH < 7.0

Potassium
- Add dosages below to each 1 l of infused fluid:
  if plasma K <3.5 mmol/l, add 40 mmol KCl
        3.5−5.5 mmol/l, add 20 mmol KCl
        >5.5 mmol/l, add no KCl

Insulin
Continuous i.v. infusion
- 5−10 U/h initially; maintenance (until able to eat), 2−4 U/h titrated against blood glucose levels, measured hourly

Intramuscular injections
- 20 U immediately, then 5−10 U/h, titrated against blood glucose levels

Other measures
- Treat precipitating cause (e.g. infection, myocardial infarction)
- Hypotension should respond to adequate fluid replacement
- Pass nasogastric tube if conscious level impaired
- Adult respiratory distress syndrome — ventilation (100% O_2, IPPV)
- Cerebral oedema — consider i.v. dexamethasone or mannitol
- Treat specific thromboembolic complications if they occur

Diabetic non-ketotic hyperosmolar coma

- Non-ketotic hyperosmolar coma is characterized by the insidious development of marked hyperglycaemia (usually >50 mmol/l), dehydration and pre-renal uraemia; significant hyperketonaemia does not develop.
- The absence of ketosis is unexplained but may be related to suppression of lipolysis by hyperosmolarity, or a reduced catabolic hormone response.
- Two-thirds of cases occur in subjects with previously undiagnosed cases of diabetes. Infection, diuretic treatment, and drinking glucose-rich beverages may all be precipitating factors.
- The condition usually affects middle-aged or elderly patients and carries a mortality of over 30%.

- Treatment involves rehydration, insulin therapy and electrolyte replacement in a manner similar to that used for diabetic ketoacidosis.

Lactic acidosis

- Severe lactic acidosis in diabetic patients (type B) occurs as a feature of ketoacidosis (in about 15% of cases) and as a rare complication of metformin therapy.
- When associated with ketoacidosis, lactic acidosis resolves with standard treatment of the ketoacidosis; that due to other causes is treated by intravenous sodium bicarbonate.
- Sodium dichloroacetate, which lowers lactate by stimulating pyruvate dehydrogenase, is a potential new treatment for lactic acidosis, but clinical experience with this agent is limited to date.

13: Diabetic microvascular disease: its nature and causes

- The *microvascular* (microangiopathic or small-vessel) complications of diabetes include retinopathy (Fig. 13.1), nephropathy and neuropathy (Fig. 13.2), even though the contribution of microangiopathy to neuropathy is unknown.
- Microvascular complications are specific to diabetes and do not occur without long-standing hyperglycaemia. Other metabolic, environmental and genetic factors are undoubtedly involved in their pathogenesis.
- Both IDDM and NIDDM are susceptible to microvascular complications, although patients with NIDDM are older at presentation and may die of macrovascular disease before microvascular disease is advanced.
- In diabetes, the microvasculature shows both functional and structural abnormalities.

- The structural hallmark of diabetic microangiopathy is thickening of the capillary basement membrane. The main functional abnormalities include increased capillary permeability, blood flow and viscosity, and disturbed platelet function. These changes occur early in the course of diabetes and precede organ failure by many years.
- The duration of diabetes and the quality of diabetic control are important determinants of microvascular disease, but because of other individual factors do not necessarily predict their development in individual patients.
- Different microvascular complications are commonly associated in individual patients, but their prevalence as a function of the duration or severity of diabetes may differ markedly.
- Over 40% of subjects with IDDM survive

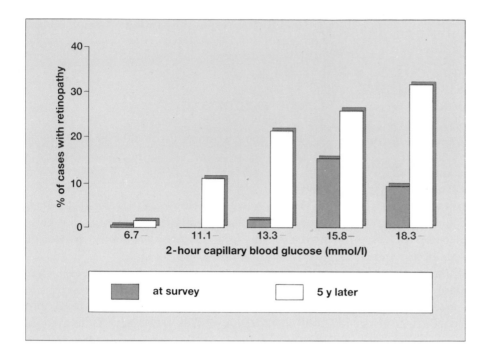

Fig. 13.1. Frequency of diabetic retinopathy in diabetic patients and those with impaired glucose tolerance in the Bedford survey, as a function of the 2-h capillary blood glucose value after a 50-g oral glucose load. Histograms show frequency at survey and 5 years later. Note that the development of retinopathy is associated with a 2-h capillary blood glucose value>11.1 mmol/l.

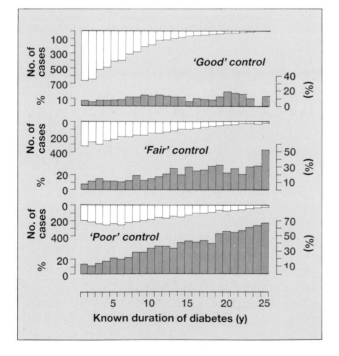

Fig. 13.2. Prevalence of diabetic neuropathy as a function of duration of diabetes in patients with good, fair and poor control. Clinical and biochemical data were collected annually from 4398 cases, over a 25-year period.

for more than 40 years, half of them without developing any significant microvascular complications.

The biochemistry of diabetic complications

• The mechanisms by which hyperglycaemia and independent risk factors (including acute cellular metabolic changes and long-term changes in stable macromolecules) interact to cause diabetic complications are summarized in Fig. 13.3.

• In insulin-independent tissues such as nerve, the renal glomerulus, lens and retina, hyperglycaemia causes elevated tissue glucose levels. The enzyme aldose reductase catalyses reduction of glucose to its polyol, sorbitol, which is subsequently converted to fructose (Fig. 13.4).

• Sorbitol does not easily cross cell membranes and its accumulation may cause damage by osmotic effects (e.g. in the lens) and altered redox state of pyridine nucleotides.

• In addition, increased sorbitol production is partly responsible for tissue depletion of myoinositol, a molecule structurally related to glucose. Hyperglycaemia itself also inhibits myoinositol uptake into cells.

• Animal studies indicate that tissue myoinositol depletion may cause abnormalities in peripheral nerve function; myoinositol is a precursor of phosphatidylinositol, the turnover of which activates Na^+-K^+-ATPase via diacylglycerol

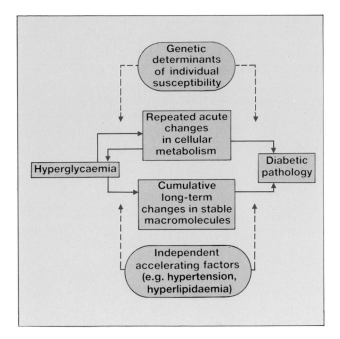

Fig. 13.3. Schematic representation of the mechanisms by which hyperglycaemia and independent risk factors interact to cause diabetic complications.

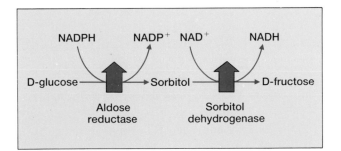

Fig. 13.4. The sorbitol (polyol) pathway. Glucose increases in insulin-independent tissues in response to hyperglycaemia and is converted to sorbitol by the enzyme aldose reductase. The accumulation of sorbitol in cells may contribute to diabetic complications by causing osmotic damage (in the lens), altering the redox state and depleting tissue myoinositol levels (thought to cause abnormalities of peripheral nerve function).

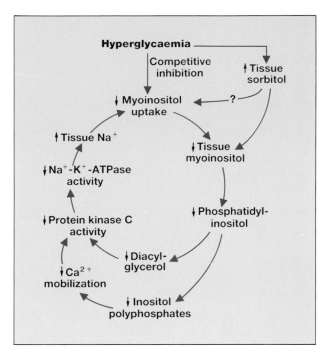

Fig. 13.5. A simplified scheme which shows some possible ways in which myoinositol depletion is involved in diabetic nerve damage. Tissue myoinositol is a precursor of phosphatidylinositol. Lowered levels of the latter depress Na^+-K^+-ATPase activity and thus slow nerve conduction velocity.

production and thus stimulation of protein kinase C (Fig. 13.5).
● Lowered Na^+-K^+-ATPase activity probably causes increased intracellular Na^+ concentrations and slows nerve conduction velocity.
● Early glycosylation products form on proteins as glucose becomes attached to amino groups. These Schiff base adducts then undergo Amadori rearrangement to form stable products analogous to glycated haemoglobin (Fig. 13.6). Such glycosylation may affect the function of a number of proteins and be partly responsible for free radical-mediated damage in diabetes.
● In long-lived molecules, early glycosylation products slowly and irreversibly form complex cross-linkings called advanced glycosylation end-products (AGE).
● Pathological consequences of AGE cross-linking include covalent binding of proteins (e.g. low density lipoprotein, albumin and IgG) to vessel walls; crosslinking of matrix components in vessel walls causing resistance to enzymatic degradation; and disturbed three-dimensional structure and altered binding of anionic proteoglycans which influence charge on the vessel wall and its interaction with bloodborne protein.

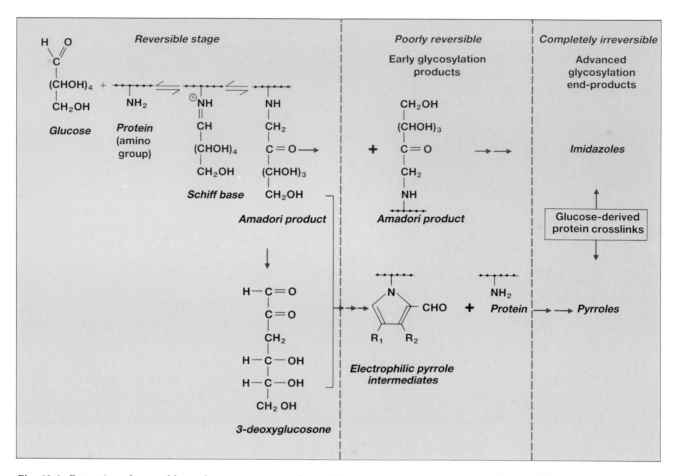

Fig. 13.6. Formation of reversible, early non-enzymatic glycosylation products on proteins and of irreversible advanced glycosylation end-products (AGE). Through a complex series of chemical reactions, Amadori products can form families of imidazole-based and pyrrole-based glucose-derived cross-links. AGE cross-links on long-lived molecules such as collagen may cause alteration of structure and function in tissues such as the vessel wall.

14: Special groups

Diabetes in childhood and adolescence

- Over 95% of cases of diabetes in childhood are due to IDDM, which has a peak age of onset of about 12 years. Principal causes of diabetes mellitus in childhood are described in Table 14.1.
- IDDM presents in children with classical symptoms, including polyuria and nocturia (often with enuresis), polydipsia, weight loss and malaise (Table 14.2). Non-specific presentations include growth failure and abdominal pain. Symptoms are usually present for a few days and occasionally up to several weeks.
- With the support of home visits by the diabetes specialist nurse, newly presenting diabetic children who are not ketotic need only a short hospital admission to begin insulin treatment and learn first aid knowledge of diabetes. Full education

Table 14.1. Principal causes of diabetes mellitus in childhood.

Insulin-dependent diabetes mellitus (IDDM) — over 95% of cases

Maturity-onset diabetes of the young (MODY)

Secondary diabetes:
- Chromosomal abnormalities: Down's syndrome
  Turner's syndrome
  Klinefelter's syndrome

- Inherited disorders: Prader–Willi syndrome
  Laurence–Moon–Biedl syndrome
  DIDMOAD syndrome

  Leprechaunism
  Lipodystrophy } with insulin
  Ataxia-telangiectasia } resistance
  Rabson–Mendenhall syndrome }
  Cystic fibrosis }
  Cystinosis } with pancreatic damage
  Thalassaemia }

- Postpancreatectomy

Table 14.2. Presenting symptoms of IDDM in childhood.

- Polyuria, including nocturia and incontinence
- Thirst and polydipsia
- Weight loss
- Growth failure (falling below height and weight centiles)
- Increased appetite, especially for carbohydrate-rich foods
- Abdominal pains and vomiting
- Blurred vision
- Muscle cramps
- Infections: (a) boils, urinary tract infections
  (b) genital or perineal candidiasis
- Behavioural disturbance, poor school performance
- Inability to concentrate
- Tiredness, lack of energy
- Ketoacidosis: (a) acidotic (Kussmaul) breathing
  (b) protracted vomiting
  (c) dehydration and postural hypotension
  (d) disturbance of consciousness
  (e) coma

---

and dietary instruction can be given gradually over the following weeks and months.
- Initial insulin dosages average 0.5 U/kg/day but are very variable. Many children show a temporary fall in insulin requirements during the first few months of treatment. This 'honeymoon period', due to transient recovery of B-cell function following reduction of hyperglycaemia, generally lasts a few months.
- Most children eventually need twice-daily insulin injections as their daytime activities become prolonged. Two-thirds of the total daily dosage may be given before breakfast and one-third before the evening meal. Biphasic, premixed insulin preparations may be useful in some cases. 'Pen' devices may help compliance with multiple injection regimens.
- Insulin injection sites should be rotated. The child should gradually be encouraged to inject itself, with no age set for the child to become independent.
- Insulin dosages should be adjusted according to glycaemic control, using self-monitored blood glucose values and HbA$_1$, and in the longer term, by growth rate and pubertal development. Diet and exercise are also important in improving glycaemic control. Physiological and behavioural changes at puberty often disturb diabetic control.
- Dietary recommendations for children with IDDM are as for adults. Foods rich in complex carbohydrate and fibre should be encouraged, whereas fat and simple sugars should be avoided.
- Exercise-induced hypoglycaemia can often be prevented by planned reductions in insulin dosage before exercise, together with extra long-acting carbohydrate (biscuits, chocolate) taken if blood glucose is less than 4 mmol/l before exercise. As for all children, sport and exercise should be encouraged.
- Intercurrent illnesses frequently cause hyperglycaemia and occasionally hypoglycaemia. Insulin must *never* be stopped and often needs to be increased. Blood glucose levels must be monitored frequently; hypoglycaemia may be controlled by sugar-rich fluids. Medical assistance is needed if symptoms last more than 12 hours, blood glucose persistently exceeds 22 mmol/l, ketonuria appears, or vomiting or diarrhoea develop.

• Adequately treated diabetes generally has little effect on growth, development, school attendance, academic performance or sporting and other activities.

• Many diabetic children do not comply fully with their management. Compliance will often be improved by providing flexible and considerate advice and is often damaged by criticism from parents or the diabetic care team.

• Diabetic ketoacidosis still carries a high morbidity and mortality in childhood. Presentation includes both classical and non-specific symptoms (Table 14.3). Important causes include intercurrent infection, omission of insulin and poor diabetic education.

• The management of diabetic ketoacidosis in children is summarized in Table 14.4, and the method of fluid replacement is outlined in Fig. 14.1.

• Cerebral oedema remains a significant cause of death from ketoacidosis in childhood. It is unexplained, but acute changes in osmolality — perhaps due to over-rapid delivery of fluid (hypotonic saline and bicarbonate have been implicated) — insulin level and a sudden glycaemic fall may contribute. Clinically significant cerebral oedema causes headache and a deterioration in conscious level due to brain herniation, sometimes with papilloedema. Computerized tomographic (CT) scanning confirms the diagnosis. Intravenous mannitol or dexamethasone, given within 10 minutes of brain herniation, may sometimes reduce intracranial pressure.

• Hypoglycaemic symptoms in diabetic children vary considerably but may include faintness, hunger, sweating, abdominal pain and irritability or aggression (Fig. 14.2). Profound and prolonged neuroglycopenia may cause fitting and unconsciousness and occasionally death. There is no firm evidence that repeated mild or moderate hypoglycaemia causes permanent brain damage.

• Children with diabetes for several years may develop features of microvascular disease. These are normally subclinical, although 'malignant' microangiopathy with rapidly deteriorating retinopathy may appear in late adolescence following long-standing diabetes.

Table 14.3. Features of diabetic ketoacidosis in children.

• Polyuria, nocturia, incontinence
• Thirst, polydipsia
• Abdominal pain
• Vomiting
• Acidotic (Kussmaul) breathing, smell of ketones on breath
• Dehydration, hypotension, collapse
• Disturbed consciousness
• Coma

Table 14.4. Management of diabetic ketoacidosis in children following urgent hospital admission.

Fluid replacement:
• Volumes (see Fig. 14.1)
• Isotonic saline; dextrose-saline or 5% dextrose when blood glucose <10 mmol/l
• Consider bicarbonate if arterial blood pH <7.0
• Consider plasma or plasma expander (25 ml/kg) initially if severe hypotension and coma are present

Potassium replacement:
• Generally 20 mmol per litre intravenous fluid
• Adjust according to plasma potassium (or ECG)

Insulin replacement:
• Continuous intravenous infusion, initially 0.1 U/kg/h
• Adjust by blood glucose monitoring

Other measures:
• Blood glucose monitoring, hourly until stable
• Fluid balance monitoring
• Plasma urea and electrolytes monitoring, 3-hourly until stable
• Arterial blood gases and pH monitoring if acidotic or hypoxaemic
• Consider oxygen; review need for intubation and ventilation
• ECG monitoring, if arrhythmias or electrolyte disturbances develop
• Nasogastric intubation, if persistent vomiting or gastric stasis occur
• Urinary catheterization, if retention or apparent oliguria develop
• If cerebral oedema suspected:
  (a) avoid fluid overload and the use of hypotonic solutions
  (b) consider intravenous mannitol or dexamethasone

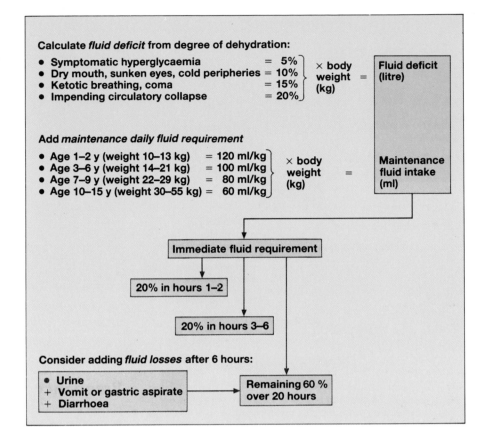

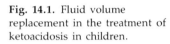

Fig. 14.1. Fluid volume replacement in the treatment of ketoacidosis in children.

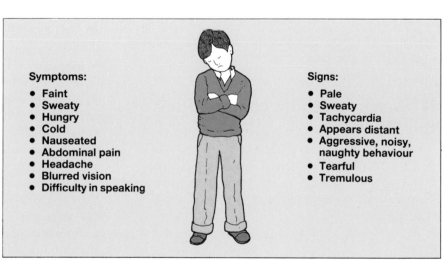

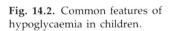

Fig. 14.2. Common features of hypoglycaemia in children.

• At least 70% of diabetic children will escape significant complications and will live long and relatively healthy lives.

• Care of diabetic children and adolescents is best delivered by a specific children's diabetic care team, comprising medical and nursing staff, a diabetes specialist sister, dietitian, social worker and paediatric psychiatrist or psychologist.

• An integrated care team is best equipped to deal with both the physiological and psycho-

logical factors which have been suggested to influence blood glucose control in children with diabetes mellitus (Fig. 14.3).

• Children with diabetes of several years' standing should be reviewed annually, with checks of blood pressure, fundi and albuminuria.

• Diabetic camps and activity holidays are greatly enjoyed by diabetic children and often help to reinforce practical and theoretical aspects of diabetic education. However, glycaemic control

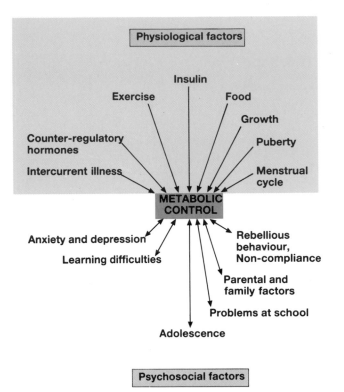

Fig. 14.3. Some factors suggested to influence blood glucose control in children with diabetes mellitus.

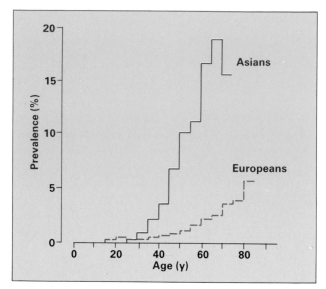

Fig. 14.4. Prevalence of known diabetes in Asians and Europeans in Southall, West London.

and ability to cope with diabetes are not apparently improved in the long term.

Diabetes in ethnic communities of the UK

- The prevalence of diabetes (mainly NIDDM) in British Asians is high — about 20% of subjects aged 60 years or more are known to have diabetes (Fig. 14.4).
- Presentation is at an earlier age than in Europeans.
- Although comparably prone to complications, the large number of Asian patients and the long exposure to diabetes may result in high future morbidity and mortality in this population.
- The cause of the high prevalence is unknown, but genetic factors are probably important.
- Similar problems may exist within the UK Afro-Caribbean community, but few data are available at present.

Pregnancy in diabetic patients

- In the absence of increased insulin administration, glycaemic control worsens during pregnancy; possible causes include tissue metabolic effects of the pregnancy hormones and resistance to insulin, and impaired insulin secretion.
- Mortality of the diabetic mother is now minimal; although there are no precise figures, it is probably slightly higher than in the general population.
- Retinopathy may worsen during pregnancy, perhaps because of the sudden improvement in metabolic control. This complication should be assessed and treated, preferably before pregnancy. Nephropathy also worsens during pregnancy and the nephrotic syndrome may develop.
- Perinatal mortality for diabetic pregnancies has improved vastly in the last 50 years but varies widely from country to country, with the standard of living and general (non-diabetic) perinatal mortality. In the UK in 1980, the general perinatal mortality was 14 per 1000 births and that for diabetic pregnancies 56 per 1000 births.
- The major causes of perinatal mortality are stillbirths (about one-half of the cases), congenital malformations (3 times higher than in the general population) and to a lesser extent, the respiratory distress syndrome (RDS), especially in babies born prematurely.

• Malformations are possibly caused by maternal hyperglycaemia and the associated metabolic perturbations in the first trimester, at the time of organogenesis — emphasizing the need for strict glycaemic control in the first 10 weeks of pregnancy.

• Babies of diabetic mothers are heavier and longer (macrosomia) than those of non-diabetic mothers, a response to increased nutrient supply to the fetus and hypersecretion of insulin by the fetal islets (Figs 14.5, 14.6). Macrosomia may lead to dystocia.

• Neonatal problems include increased proneness to RDS and jaundice (diseases of prematurity), hypoglycaemia (continued hypersecretion of insulin by the B-cell), polycythaemia (due to relative fetal hypoxia) and hypocalcaemia (hyposecretion of parathyroid hormone).

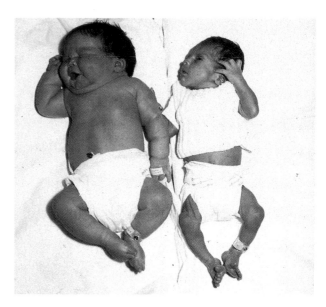

Fig. 14.6. Left: a macrosomic baby born to a diabetic mother. Right: a normal baby born to a non-diabetic mother.

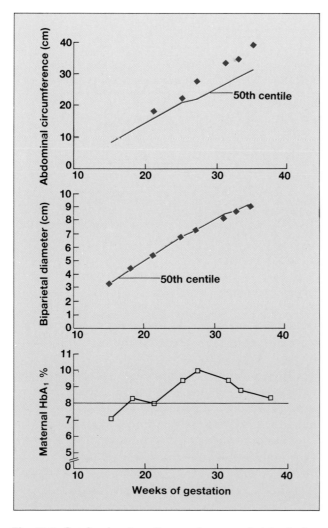

Fig. 14.5. Graphs showing ultrasound-measured abdominal circumference of a fetus (◆) outstripping biparietal diameter, and thus indicating macrosomia.

• The management of a diabetic pregnancy requires a team approach and starts with pre-pregnancy counselling to offer contraceptive advice, explain the risks and relative contraindications of pregnancy, treat complications and above all help the woman to achieve better glycaemic control (Tables 14.5, 14.6).

• Antenatal visits at weekly or up to monthly intervals should include assessment and management of glycaemic control, diabetic complications (including hypertension), and potential obstetric complications, especially pre-eclampsia, hydramnios and urinary tract infections (Table 14.7).

• Control may be optimized by dietary and insulin adjustments; the latter based on home glucose monitoring data. HbA$_1$ will provide a check on glycaemic control. Continuous adjustments of insulin dose will need to be made and more than two daily insulin injections may be required.

• Delivery should be after at least 38 weeks in the absence of obstetric problems. Normoglycaemia is advisable, particularly in prolonged labour, and can be provided by intravenous insulin and dextrose infusions. Vaginal delivery is preferable; the indications for caesarean section are pelvic disproportion, an abnormal uterus, placenta praevia, marked macrosomia and presentations other than cephalic.

• Gestational diabetes mellitus (GDM) is diabetes which presents in pregnancy, commonly in the middle of the second trimester. The frequency is

---

Do the prospective parents understand the risks?
- To the mother:
  - Diabetes increases the risk of death slightly compared with the general pregnant population
  - Active retinopathy, nephropathy, and heart disease may get worse
  - Caesarean section is much more likely

- To the baby:
  - Diabetes increases the risk of death about three-fold
  - Malformations are 3 times commoner and more often multiple
  - Serious neonatal complications are commoner
  - Long-term risk of developing diabetes is slightly increased

- To the father:
  - The need to provide additional care to mother and baby

Does the mother understand what a diabetic pregnancy involves?
- Close supervision with frequent antenatal visits
- Home blood glucose monitoring several times per day
- Two or more insulin injections per day
- Careful attention to diet
- Stopping smoking and drinking alcohol

Do the prospective parents need:
- Contraceptive advice?
- Genetic counselling?

Table 14.5. Key facts for prepregnancy counselling. The risks are based on survey data and they should be substantially reduced if the advice is given and heeded.

Optimize glycaemic control	*Targets*
Self-monitoring and education	Preprandial BG 3–5 mmol/l
Adjust insulin if necessary	Postprandial BG <10 mmol/l
Check diet	HbA$_1$ in non-diabetic range
Check HbA$_1$	

Assess diabetic complications
Retinopathy (visual acuity, fundoscopy)
Nephropathy (proteinuria, blood urea, creatinine)
Vascular disease (hypertension, ischaemic heart and peripheral vascular disease)
Autonomic neuropathy (vomiting)

Discourage smoking and drinking alcohol

Obstetric assessment

Table 14.6. Initial evaluation of the pregnant diabetic woman.

Table 14.7. Subsequent evaluation of the pregnant diabetic woman in the combined diabetic-obstetric clinic.

Optimize glycaemic control (as above)

Assess diabetic complications

Check for obstetric complications
Pre-eclampsia
Hydramnios
Urinary tract infections

Assess fetal growth by ultrasound examination
Crown–rump measurement in first trimester
  (confirm dates)
17 weeks: detailed survey for major malformations
19–20 weeks: detailed examination of fetal heart
Regular head and abdominal girth measurements to
  assess growth progress and to detect macrosomia

---

between 1 and 2% of pregnancies, with an increased risk in the obese and those with a family history of diabetes.
- GDM is rarely symptomatic and can only be detected by screening (Fig. 14.7). Although there is no consensus, screening at 28 weeks detects the majority of GDM. A random blood glucose of >6.0 mmol/l or a value >8.0 mmol/l 1 hour after a 75-g oral glucose tolerance test, is suggestive of GDM. A full oral glucose tolerance test should then be performed to confirm the diagnosis.
- Management of GDM includes assessment of diet and appropriate adjustments to reduce obesity. Adequate glycaemia is not achieved in about one-third of the women; insulin must then be

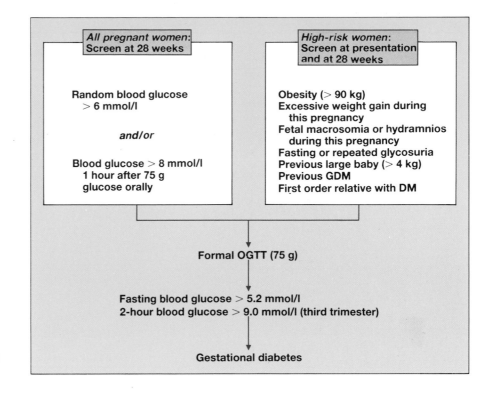

Fig. 14.7. Screening and diagnosis of gestational diabetes.

added and postpregnancy follow-up is desirable to ensure that diabetes has resolved.

Contraception in diabetic patients

• Most diabetic women can safely have children, but pregnancy is contraindicated by advanced nephropathy, ischaemic heart disease, severe symptomatic autonomic neuropathy and untreated proliferative retinopathy (Table 14.8). Sterilization may be indicated in some cases.

• Contraceptive advice must be carefully tailored to the couple's needs. The main contraceptive methods available to diabetic women are considered in Table 14.9, and the relative chances of pregnancy with various contraceptive methods are shown in Table 14.10.

• Combined oral contraceptive pills containing high-dose oestrogens aggravate glycaemic and lipaemic profiles, and are not recommended in diabetic women. Newer, low oestrogen-dose pills have very high success rates and few metabolic side-effects, and are suitable in young patients with no diabetic complications or risk factors for vascular disease.

Table 14.8. Contraindications to pregnancy in diabetic women.

• Advanced nephropathy
  — creatinine clearance <40 ml/min
  — heavy proteinuria or nephrotic syndrome
  — associated severe hypertension
• Significant coronary heart disease
• Proliferative retinopathy, if left untreated
• Autonomic neuropathy with severe hyperemesis

• Progestogen-only pills have no adverse metabolic effects and are effective if used regularly. They may cause menstrual disturbance, including amenorrhoea.

• Intra-uterine devices have no metabolic side-effects but have a generally higher failure rate and may carry an increased risk of infection in diabetic women.

• Mechanical methods (condom or diaphragm) have high failure rates unless used carefully and are not recommended if pregnancy is contraindicated.

Table 14.9. Main contraceptive methods available for diabetic women.

Methods	Adverse effects on:		Thrombo-embolic risk	Other comments
	Glycaemia	Lipidaemia		
Oral contraceptive pill:				
Combined { high-dose E + P	+	+	+	Avoid combined pills if other risk factors for coronary disease are present: smoking, hypertension, hyperlipidaemia, positive family history
low-dose E + P	–	±	±	
low-dose E + P, triphasic	–	±	±	
Progestogen only ('mini-pill')	–	–	–	Menstrual irregularity; use other contraceptive method if more than one pill missed (e.g. by omission, vomiting or diarrhoea)
Intra-uterine contraceptive device	–	–	–	Possibly increased risk of pelvic infection; relatively high failure rate
Barrier methods (± spermicide)	–	–	–	High failure rate; avoid if pregnancy absolutely contra-indicated

Notes: E, oestrogen; high dose $\geq 50\,\mu g$ of ethinyl oestradiol or equivalent; low dose $\leq 30\,\mu g$. P, progestogen.

Method	If method is used correctly	General experience of method
No method	80	80
Withdrawal	20	40
Rhythm method	10	25
Spermicides	10	20
Diaphragm	5	10
Condom	5	10
IUCD	4	4
Contraceptive pill	<1	2
Vasectomy	<1	<1
Tubal sterilization	<1	<1

Table 14.10. The chances of pregnancy with various contraceptive methods: the number of women who will become pregnant for each 100 couples who use the method for 1 year is indicated.

15: Living with diabetes: intercurrent events and surgery in diabetic patients

Surgery in diabetic patients

• Surgical stress suppresses insulin release and stimulates counter-regulatory hormone secretion, increasing catabolism overall; in insulin-deficient diabetic patients, hyperglycaemia and ketosis may result.

• Hypoglycaemia due to excessive insulin or sulphonylurea treatment in starved patients is the other major hazard of surgery.

• A system of preoperative assessment of the diabetic patient is recommended (Table 15.1).

• Successful management of surgery in diabetic patients requires a simple and safe procedure which is fully understood by all staff (Table 15.2, Fig. 15.1).

• Long-acting sulphonylureas or insulins should be changed for shorter-acting agents some days before surgery, to reduce the risk of hypoglycaemia.

• Well-controlled NIDDM patients undergoing minor surgery only require close glycaemic monitoring. Poorly controlled NIDDM patients, or those requiring major surgery, should be treated as for IDDM.

Table 15.1. Preoperative assessment of the diabetic patient requiring surgery.

• Assess glycaemic control
• Adjust diabetic treatment as necessary to optimize glycaemic control; substitute shorter-acting preparations for chlorpropamide or ultralente
• Arrange other investigations if needed, e.g. chest X-ray, electrocardiogram, renal function
• Arrange for surgery in morning if possible
• Liaise with anaesthetist

Table 15.2. Principles of diabetes management during surgery.

Insulin-treated patient (mostly IDDM)	Non-insulin-treated patient
Assume patient has no insulin reserves	Assume patient has limited insulin reserves
↓	↓
Intravenous insulin and glucose needed for all grades of surgery	Intravenous insulin and glucose needed for major surgery only. Otherwise observation alone is sufficient

1 **Ensure satisfactory preoperative control. Operate in morning if possible**

2 **Liaise with anaesthetist**

3 **Omit breakfast, and insulin or oral hypoglycaemic drug, on morning of surgery**

4 **Non-insulin treated diabetic patients, having non-major surgery, need observation only. Chart 2-hourly glucose reagent strips on day of surgery. Patients taking oral hypoglycaemic drugs can restart those with next meal**

5 **Glucose-potassium-insulin ('GKI') is used in all other cases, i.e. (a) all insulin-treated diabetics; and (b) major surgery in non-insulin treated diabetics**

(i) At 8–9 a.m. on morning of surgery, start GKI infusion:

500 ml 10% dextrose
+15 U short-acting insulin } Infuse 5-hourly (100 ml/h)
+10 mmol KCl

(ii) Check blood glucose 2-hourly initially and aim for 6–11 mmol/l.
If > 11 mmol/l, change to GKI with 20 U insulin
If < 6mmol/l, change to GKI with 10 U insulin
Continue to adjust as necessary
(iii) Continue GKI until patients eat, then revert to usual treatment. If GKI is prolonged (> 24 h), check electrolytes daily for possible Na$^+$ or K$^+$ abnormalities

Fig. 15.1 A simple protocol for diabetes management during surgery.

• IDDM patients require continuous administration of both insulin and glucose during surgery, ideally with potassium to prevent hypokalaemia. The standard cocktail is 15 U short-acting insulin plus 10 mmol KCl in 500 ml of 10% dextrose, given intravenously at 100 ml/h (Table 15.3). The insulin dosage should be changed in case of hyper- or hypoglycaemia.

• Open-heart surgery requires higher rates of insulin delivery because of glucose-rich solutions and inotropes used during bypass, and the metabolic effects of hypothermia.

Travel

• Diabetes is not a bar to travel, even over long distances, but careful planning, adequate supplies of medication and sensible self-monitoring are essential.

• Patients must be fully instructed in what to do during diarrhoea, vomiting or other intercurrent illness.

• Insulin can be kept safely at warm room temperature for at least 1 month.

• Extended days during long westward air journeys often require an additional dose of short-acting insulin followed by a meal.

Driving and diabetes

• Diabetes (especially IDDM) presents several potential hazards to the driver, although there is little evidence that diabetic drivers suffer more traffic accidents than other drivers.

• In the UK, all drivers are legally required to notify diabetes to the Driver and Vehicle Licensing Centre and to their own insurance company.

• Diabetic drivers in the UK can hold Public Service or Heavy Goods Vehicle licences, but in practice those treated with insulin are barred from driving vehicles which carry passengers.

• Hypoglycaemia must be avoided while driving by careful planning and blood glucose testing; a supply of glucose must be kept in the car.

• The minimum legal requirement for a driver's vision (reading a standard number plate at 23 m; roughly 6/10) does not take account of many visual problems caused by diabetes, which require separate assessment.

• All diabetic patients must be asked if they drive; those who do must be given appropriate advice (Table 15.4).

Employment, insurance, smoking and alcohol

• Insulin-treated diabetic patients are barred from only a few occupations where hypoglycaemia poses particular hazards to themselves or others (e.g. public transport, armed forces).

• Non-insulin-treated patients without complications should enjoy the same job prospects as non-diabetic people.

• Special life insurance policies are available for diabetic people.

• The risks of developing coronary heart and other macrovascular disease are markedly increased by diabetes and by smoking, and almost

1 Standard GKI 'cocktail'	500 ml 10% dextrose (glucose) solution + 15 U short-acting insulin + 10 mmol KCl	Infuse over 5 h (100 ml/h)
2 Sliding scale control	Measure blood glucose with strip 1–2 hourly initially: 6–11 mmol/l → standard GKI cocktail >11 mmol/l → GKI containing 20 U insulin <6 mmol/l → GKI containing 10 U insulin Continue 5-U adjustments as necessary	

Table 15.3. The glucose–potassium–insulin or 'GKI' infusion system.

Notes: (1) Any short-acting insulin can be used, e.g. Humulin S, Velosulin, Actrapid. (2) The frequency of monitoring can usually be reduced later. (3) In practice, alterations in the standard GKI infusion are not often needed; if so, the current infusion bag should be taken down and a new bag (containing the altered insulin dosage) substituted.

Table 15.4. Advice to diabetic drivers.

- Inform the licensing authority (UK: DVLC) and motor insurer (these are legal requirements in many countries)
- Always keep a supply of glucose in the car
- Avoid long journeys without rest periods and meals, and check blood glucose levels frequently
- If hypoglycaemic, stop driving and leave the driver's seat
- Do not drive if eyesight deteriorates suddenly (e.g. after vitreous haemorrhage), or if corrected visual acuity is less than 6/12 in both eyes

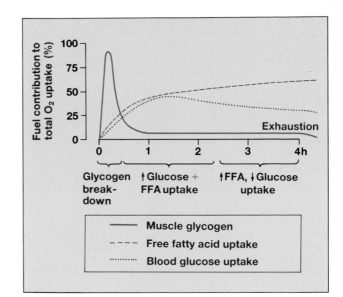

Fig. 15.2. The relative contributions of muscle glycogen breakdown and uptake of blood-borne glucose and non-esterified fatty acids to fuel utilization at various stages of prolonged exercise in normal man. The exercise intensity corresponds to 30% of maximal.

certainly further increased by smoking and diabetes together. Diabetic patients must be strongly discouraged from smoking.

- Alcohol readily provokes hypoglycaemia in diabetic patients. Daily alcohol intake should not exceed three equivalents (e.g. three small glasses of wine) for diabetic men or two equivalents for diabetic women (Table 15.5).

Exercise and diabetes mellitus

Due to its hypoglycaemic effect, exercise has traditionally been recommended as an important component of diabetic treatment. In recent years, much new information has accumulated regarding the beneficial and possible adverse effects of exercise for diabetic patients. This section focuses on the effects of acute exercise and physical training in diabetes and outlines practical recommendations for exercise.

- Energy for muscular work is derived initially from the breakdown of muscle glycogen and later from circulating glucose and non-esterified fatty acids; muscle uptake of glucose may increase 20-fold during exercise, due to increased blood flow and glucose delivery and to enhanced glucose transporter activity (Fig. 15.2).

Table 15.5. The British Diabetic Association's recommendations regarding alcohol consumption by diabetic patients. One equivalent (or unit) = a single measure of spirits, a small glass of wine, or a half-pint of beer.

- Maximum daily intake = three equivalents for men, or two equivalents for women
- Never take alcohol without food, or before driving
- Include calorie contents of drinks in weight-reducing diets; avoid sweet wines, liqueurs and 'mixers'
- Patients taking sulphonylureas should limit their alcohol intake, and those with neuropathic symptoms or hypertriglyceridaemia should abstain completely

- Hepatic glucose production (mainly from glycogenolysis) normally rises to meet increased glucose demands but ultimately may be unable to match glucose consumption; normal people may become hypoglycaemic after 2–3 h of strenuous exercise without caloric intake.
- During prolonged exercise, a normal subject's insulin secretion declines and release of counter-regulatory hormones increases.

Effects of exercise in IDDM patients

Different considerations become important in IDDM because of the lack of regulation of insulin entry into the circulation.

- In IDDM, glycaemic changes during exercise depend largely on blood insulin levels and therefore on insulin administration and absorption; absorption may be accelerated by exercising an injected limb. Hyperinsulinaemia causes hypoglycaemia, which may persist for many hours as muscle glycogen stores are replenished. Hypoinsulinaemia, combined with counter-regulatory hormone excesses, leads rapidly to hyperglycaemia. These different influences are summarized in Table 15.6 and Fig. 15.3.

Table 15.6. Factors determining glycaemic response to acute exercise in IDDM patients.

Blood glucose decreases if:
- Hyperinsulinaemia exists during exercise
- Exercise is prolonged (>30–60 min) or intensive
- >3 h have elapsed since the preceding meal
- No extra snacks are taken before or during the exercise

Blood glucose remains unchanged if:
- Exercise is short
- Plasma insulin concentration is normal
- Appropriate snacks are taken before and during exercise

Blood glucose increases if:
- Hypoinsulinaemia exists during exercise
- Exercise is strenous
- Excessive carbohydrate is taken before or during exercise

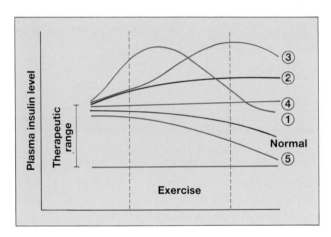

Fig. 15.3. Plasma insulin levels may vary widely during exercise in insulin-treated diabetic patients, whereas normal subjects show a steady decline during prolonged exercise. *Hyperinsulinaemia* and hypoglycaemia may occur when the peak action of short-acting (1) or intermediate-acting (2) insulin occurs during exercise or if exercise itself accelerates absorption from an injected leg (3). Steady insulin concentrations (4) may occur during CSII or after intermediate-acting insulin injection. Declining levels (5) and *hypoinsulinaemia* occur when the previous injections are exhausted.

- Insulin-treated IDDM patients can reduce the risks of hypoglycaemia during acute exercise by taking 20–40 g extra carbohydrate before and hourly during exercise and/or by reducing pre-exercise insulin dosages by 30–50%. Glycaemia should be monitored during and after exercise; post-exercise hypoglycaemia may be delayed until the following day.

Effects of exercise in NIDDM patients

- In NIDDM, exercise increases peripheral glucose uptake but also decreases endogenous insulin secretion; hypoglycaemia is therefore rare and extra carbohydrate is not generally required (Fig. 15.4). However, sulphonylureas may cause hypoglycaemia during exercise.

Benefits of exercise and practical advice for patients

- Long-term physical training in normal and diabetic people increases insulin sensitivity and in diabetic subjects may improve glycaemic and lipaemic profiles. Physical training in youth may also protect against the subsequent development of NIDDM.

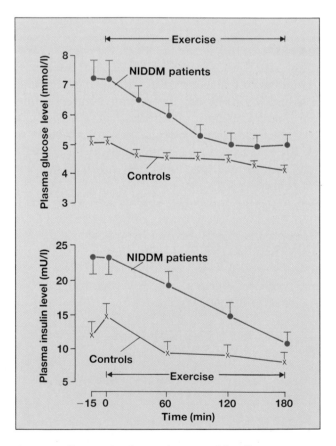

Fig. 15.4. Changes in plasma glucose and insulin concentrations during prolonged exercise in non-obese NIDDM patients. The exercise (30–35% of maximal) was performed after an overnight fast. The fall in endogenous insulin secretion diminishes the risk of hypoglycaemia during exercise in NIDDM.

• Diabetic patients can undertake most sports, but insulin treatment contraindicates those where hypoglycaemia would be dangerous, and patients with proliferative retinopathy or severe arterial disease should not take strenuous exercise.
• Guidelines for exercise in IDDM and NIDDM are suggested in Tables 15.7–15.9.

Infection

• Infection impairs glycaemic control in diabetic patients and is one of the commoner identified precipitating factors for diabetic ketoacidosis.

Table 15.7. Cautions and advice regarding exercise in diabetes.

Contraindications
Insulin treatment: sports where hypoglycaemia would be dangerous (e.g. diving, climbing, single-handed sailing, motor racing)
Proliferative retinopathy: strenuous exercise (risk of possible haemorrhage)

Cautions
Cardiovascular disease (especially in NIDDM)
Peripheral neuropathy (risk of injury to feet)

General advice
Take exercise regularly, daily if possible
Strenuous exertion is not necessary; even regular walking has metabolic benefits
Tailor exercise schedules to the patient's individual needs and physical fitness

---

Table 15.8. Guidelines for exercise in IDDM.

• Monitor glycaemia before, during and after exercise
• Avoid hypoglycaemia during exercise by:
  — starting exercise 1–2 h after a meal
  — taking 20–40 g extra carbohydrate before and hourly during exercise
  — avoiding heavy exercise during peak insulin action
  — using non-exercising sites for insulin injection
  — reducing pre-injection insulin dosages by 30–50% if necessary
• After prolonged exercise, monitor glycaemia and take extra carbohydrate to avoid delayed hypoglycaemia

---

Table 15.9. Guidelines for exercise in NIDDM.

• Hypoglycaemia is unlikely during exercise and extra carbohydrate is therefore generally unnecessary
• Exercise used to reduce weight should be combined with dietary measures
• Exercise should be part of the daily schedule

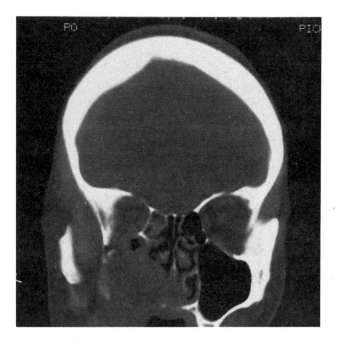

Fig. 15.5. CT scan showing rhinocerebral mucormycosis in a diabetic patient. The right maxillary sinus is filled and there is invasion of the floor of the orbit and the turbinates.

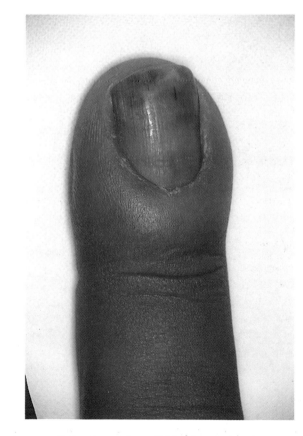

Fig. 15.6. Bolstering of the nail-fold due to chronic paronychia involving *Candida*.

• The presence of diabetes impairs several aspects of phagocyte function, including cell movement, phagocytosis and intracellular killing of micro-organisms; hyperglycaemia reduces oxidative killing capacity because increased glucose metabolism through the polyol pathway consumes NADPH, which is necessary to generate super-oxide radicals.

• Although diabetic patients are strikingly prone to unusual infections with rare organisms (e.g. mucoromycosis, enterococcal meningitis, osteo-myelitis), to tuberculosis and to complicated urinary tract infections, it is not clear whether their general susceptibility to infection is increased or not (Figs 15.5, 15.6).

16: Drugs and diabetes mellitus

Many drugs can affect glucose metabolism and cause hyper- or hypoglycaemia and many can also interact with the action of sulphonylurea drugs to influence diabetic control. It is important to be aware of the most important drug effects and interactions to explain and, better still, to pre-empt any drug-induced disturbances in diabetic control.

Drugs causing or exacerbating hyperglycaemia

• The major mechanisms through which drugs can induce hyperglycaemia are shown in Fig. 16.1, and the most important drugs are indicated in Table 16.1.
• Of these agents, corticosteroids are the drugs with the greatest hyperglycaemic effect. Diabetic treatment must be adjusted before starting high-dose steroid therapy: most IDDM patients require a 50% increase in insulin dosage and many NIDDM patients treated with diet or oral agents will need insulin.
• Thiazide diuretics are diabetogenic in non-diabetic and NIDDM subjects (possibly by inhibiting insulin secretion) but have no hyper-glycaemic effect in IDDM patients receiving insulin. Frusemide or other loop diuretics are not diabetogenic and are the diuretics of choice in NIDDM.

• Oral contraceptives containing low-dose oestrogen and progestogen, or progestogen alone, have no significant hyperglycaemic action and are acceptable in IDDM and probably in NIDDM and women with previous gestational diabetes. The progestogen, levonorgestrel may be diabet-ogenic.
• β_2-adrenergic agents (e.g. salbutamol, ritodrine) when given by intravenous infusion stimulate gluconeogenesis and cause hyperglycaemia.

Drugs causing or exacerbating hypoglycaemia or its symptoms

• Important examples are shown in Table 16.2.
• Of these drugs, β-blocking agents, both β_1-selective and non-selective, can mask important hypoglycaemic symptoms and should be pre-scribed cautiously in patients taking insulin or sulphonylurea drugs. However, recent evidence suggests that this effect may not be as pro-nounced as previously assumed.

Drug interactions with the sulphonylureas

• Many drugs either reduce or increase the hypoglycaemic action of the sulphonylureas (see

Table 16.1. Drugs causing or exacerbating hyperglycaemia.

System indication	Drug class and examples	Mechanisms	Effects and comments
Cardiovascular drugs	*β-adrenergic blockers*	• Inhibit insulin secretion (β_2 action) and sensitivity	• May impair glucose tolerance in NIDDM or non-diabetic people • Rarely clinically significant
	Potassium-losing diuretics: Thiazides (e.g. bendrofluazide) Thiazide-related (e.g. chlorthalidone, metolazone)	• Cause potassium depletion which may impair insulin secretion	• May impair glucose tolerance in NIDDM or non-diabetic people • Thiazides combined with β-blockers are more deleterious • No firm evidence that loop diuretics (e.g. frusemide) worsen glucose tolerance
	Vasodilator: Diazoxide	• Directly inhibits insulin secretion	• Hyperglycaemia may develop after a few injections
	Anti-arrhythmic drug: Encainide	• Unknown	• Hyperglycaemia may develop after some weeks of treatment
Respiratory system drugs	*β₂-adrenergic stimulants*: Salbutamol, terbutaline	• Increase hepatic glucose output	• Acute hyperglycaemia only with high intravenous dosages • May precipitate ketoacidosis in IDDM patients
Anti-microbial agents	Pentamidine	• Causes B-cell destruction	• Often initial hypoglycaemia • Irreversible hyperglycaemia may occur during or even weeks after treatment
	Rifampicin	• Enhances glucose absorption from gut	• Mild postprandial hyperglycaemia • Clinically unimportant
Obstetric drugs	*β₂-adrenergic stimulants*: Salbutamol, terbutaline, ritodrine	• Increase hepatic glucose output	• Acute hyperglycaemia only with high intravenous dosages • Exacerbated by dexamethasone given concurrently to accelerate fetal lung maturation

(continued on next page)

Table 16.1. Drugs causing or exacerbating hyperglycaemia (*contd*).

System indication	Drug class and examples	Mechanisms	Effects and comments
Endocrine drugs	*Glucocorticoids*: Cortisone, hydrocortisone, prednisolone, dexamethasone; also corticotrophin (ACTH)	• Postreceptor inhibition of insulin action; increase glycogenolysis and gluconeogenesis	• Dose-related hyperglycaemia • Only occurs with doses > 7.5 mg/day prednisolone or equivalent
	Oral contraceptives: Synthetic oestrogens and/or progestogens	• Postreceptor inhibition of insulin action	• Hyperglycaemia due mainly to oestrogens; some progestogens also implicated • On present evidence, sequential low-oestrogen or progestogen-only pills cause little metabolic disturbance
	Anabolic and related steroids: Oxymetholone, danazol, stanozolol	• Postreceptor inhibition of insulin action	• Impairment of glucose tolerance may result
	Growth hormone	• Postreceptor inhibition of insulin action	• Impairment of glucose tolerance may result
	Somatostatin analogues: Octreotide	• Inhibits insulin secretion; also inhibits glucagon and growth hormone secretion and glucose absorption from gut	• May worsen glucose tolerance in normal subjects; little change in NIDDM; improved in insulin-treated patients

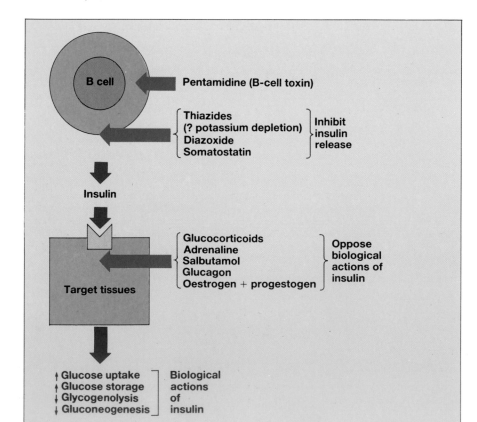

Fig. 16.1 Mechanisms by which drugs may induce hyperglycaemia.

Table 16.2. Drugs causing or exacerbating hypoglycaemia.

System indication	Drug class and examples	Mechanisms	Effects and comments
Cardiovascular drugs	*β-adrenergic blockers*	• Block catecholamine action	• Reduce some symptoms of hypoglycaemia (tremor, tachycardia) and possibly neuroglycopenia • May delay recovery from hypoglycaemia
	Anti-arrhythmic drugs: Quinidine	• Stimulates insulin secretion	• May cause hypoglycaemia, especially in overdose and in fasting or severely ill patients
	Lipid-lowering drugs: Fibrates, e.g. bezafibrate, gemfibrozil	• Reduce free fatty acid levels, so stimulate peripheral glucose utilization	• Clinically not important
Analgesics and anti-inflammatory drugs	Salicylates	• Decrease hepatic glucose output	• In high therapeutic doses or overdosage • Especially in children; often fatal in this group
	Paracetamol	• Acute hepatic necrosis reduces hepatic glucose output	• In acute overdose; often fatal
Anti-microbial agents	Quinine	• Stimulates insulin secretion	• High risk in malaria, mainly cerebral in children and in pregnancy; exaggerated in renal failure; often fatal
	Sulphamethoxazole (in co-trimoxazole)	• Stimulates insulin secretion (sulphonylurea-like action)	• In elderly patients receiving high doses • Exaggerated in renal failure
	Pentamidine	• Causes insulin release due to B-cell damage	• Hypoglycaemia during first weeks of treatment • Irreversible hyperglycaemia may follow
Miscellaneous	Ethanol	• Inhibits gluconeogenesis • Effect exaggerated if hepatic glycogen is depleted	• Especially in malnutrition • Profound hypoglycaemia may follow 2−3 h after drinking alcohol with high-glucose food or drink

Table 16.3); potential interactions must always be checked before starting other drugs in sulphonylurea-treated patients and blood glucose levels should be carefully monitored. The elderly and tightly controlled patients are at particular risk of hypoglycaemia.

Drugs and patients with diabetic complications

• Certain drugs are absolutely or relatively contraindicated in patients with certain diabetic complications. The most important examples are listed in Table 16.4.

Increased hypoglycaemic effect	Decreased hypoglycaemic effect
Sulphonylureas	
Hypoglycaemic agents (see Table 16.2)	*Hyperglycaemic agents* (see Table 16.1)
Decreased sulphonylurea clearance:	*Increased hepatic sulphonylurea clearance:*
• Azapropazone	• Alcohol (chronic intake)
• Phenylbutazone, oxyphenbutazone	• Rifampicin
• Sulphinpyrazone	• Chlorpromazine
• Sulphonamides	
• Salicylates	
• Probenecid	
• Monoamine oxidase inhibitors	
• Chloramphenicol	
• Nicoumalone	
(but not warfarin or phenindione)	
Metformin	
Cimetidine reduces renal clearance of metformin, thus raising its plasma levels and increasing the risks of toxicity	

Table 16.3. Drugs interacting with oral hypoglycaemic agents.

Table 16.4. Drugs requiring caution in specific diabetic complications.

Complication and drug	Problem	Action to be taken
Nephropathy Sulphonylureas	• Accumulate in renal failure; increased risk of hypoglycaemia and toxicity	• Use insulin or a sulphonylurea not cleared through the kidneys (e.g. gliquidone, gliclazide)
Metformin	• Accumulates in renal failure; increased risk of lactic acidosis	• Avoid completely
Cardiovascular disease β-adrenergic blockers	• Accentuate hypoglycaemia • May cause modest VLDL elevation	• Consider alternative antihypertensive, anti-anginal or anti-arrhythmic drugs (e.g. ACE inhibitors, calcium channel blockers)
Thiazide diuretics	• Aggravate glycaemic control in NIDDM • Exacerbate hyperlipidaemia	• Use loop diuretic or alternative anti-hypertensive drugs
Retinopathy Mydriatics (eyedrops or systemic atropinic drugs)	• In patients with rubeosis or previous eye surgery, glaucoma may be precipitated	• Seek ophthalmological advice before dilating pupils
Anticoagulants and thrombolytic drugs	• May predispose to vitreous haemorrhage in patients with proliferative changes	• Avoid if possible
Autonomic neuropathy: *Postural hypotension* Ganglion-blocking agents and vasodilators	• Aggravate postural hypotension	• Avoid, especially in the elderly
Impotence Ganglion-blocking agents β-adrenergic blockers Clonidine α-methyldopa Thiazide diuretics (?)	• Aggravate erectile failure	• Use alternative antihypertensive drugs, e.g. ACE inhibitors, calcium channel blockers or prazosin

17: Diabetic eye disease

The lesions

- The lesions of diabetic retinopathy can be grouped into those associated with background, preproliferative and proliferative retinopathy (Table 17.1).
- Background retinopathy is characterized by: capillary dilatation (later with leakage), capillary occlusion, microaneurysms, blot haemorrhages and lipid-rich hard exudates (commonly in the macular area and associated with oedema) (Figs 17.1 & 17.2).
- In preproliferative retinopathy, there are 'cotton-wool' spots (interruption of axoplasmic transport indicating retinal ischaemia — see Fig. 17.3), venous abnormalities (loops, beading and re-duplication — see Fig. 17.5), arterial abnormalities (variation of calibre, narrowing of segments and occlusion) and intraretinal microvascular abnormalities (IRMA — clusters of dilated abnormal capillaries lying within the retina — see Figs 17.3, 17.4).
- In proliferative retinopathy, new vessels arise in the periphery (Fig. 17.5) and/or on the optic disc (Fig. 17.6), eventually with a fibrous tissue covering. The visual complications are caused by vitreous retraction which leads to preretinal haemorrhage (Fig. 17.6) and vitreous haemorrhage, and to traction and detachment of the retina.
- New vessels on the optic disc are a high-risk feature as they often cause complications of haemorrhage and retinal detachment.
- Uncomplicated background retinopathy is common and in most patients remains mild for many years. Turnover of microaneurysms, haemorrhages and hard exudates is relatively rapid.
- Maculopathy is heralded by rings of hard exudates approaching the fovea.
- Maculopathy occurs mostly in NIDDM and can cause severe visual loss which is often central, with preserved peripheral navigational vision. It can be exudative, oedematous (sometimes with cystoid changes) or ischaemic (Fig. 17.7).
- Proliferative retinopathy is the commonest sight-threatening lesion in IDDM. Advanced diabetic eye disease is its end stage, defined by long-standing vitreous haemorrhage (Fig. 17.8), macular traction or detachment, or thrombotic glaucoma.
- Thrombotic glaucoma is due to new vessels and fibrous tissue proliferating in the angle of the

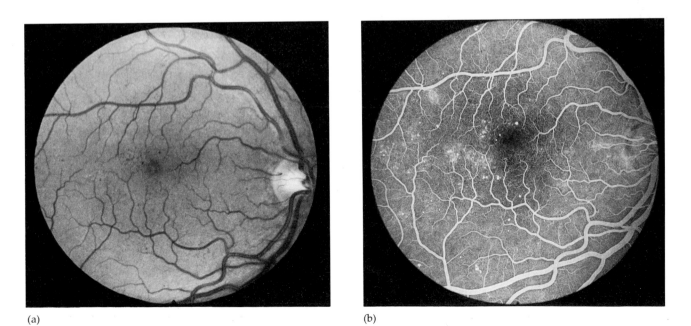

(a) (b)

Fig. 17.1. (a) From a colour photograph of the right macular area of a diabetic patient with mild retinopathy, showing only a few microaneurysms and early hard exudates. (b) Fluorescein photograph of area shown in (a). Note many more microaneurysms showing up as white dots.

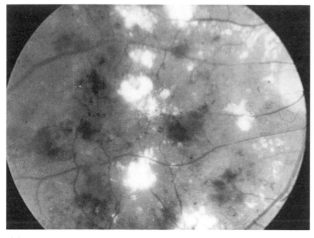

(a)

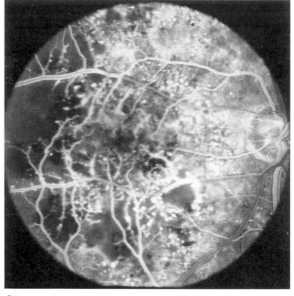

(b)

Fig. 17.2. (a) Right macular area of a patient with large blot haemorrhages and hard exudates. (b) Fluorescein angiogram of area shown in (a). Note large areas of non-perfusion and the darker areas indicating ischaemic haemorrhages between perfused and non-perfused retina (arrows).

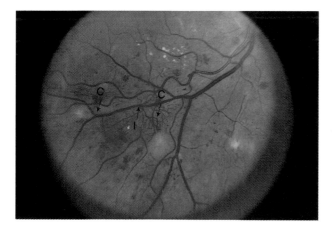

Fig. 17.3. Shows cotton-wool spots (C), IRMA (I), deep round haemorrhages and the 'empty retina' of preproliferative retinopathy.

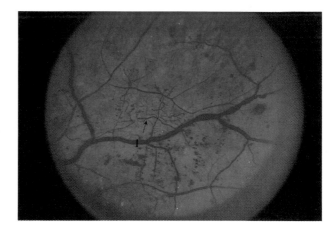

Fig. 17.4. Shows venous beading and IRMA (I) of preproliferative retinopathy.

anterior chamber, preventing drainage of the aqueous. It is associated with rubeosis iridis (neovascularization of the iris) and can cause severe pain and irreversible blindness (Fig. 17.9).
• The presence of diabetes accelerates the development of senile cataracts, by two- to threefold in patients in their 50s and 60s. Juvenile cataracts with a snowflake appearance may be precipitated acutely by a period of poor metabolic control.

Epidemiology

• Diabetes is the commonest cause of visual loss in the British working population.
• The prevalence of retinopathy increases with duration of diabetes (Fig. 17.10). In young-onset, insulin-treated diabetic patients, proliferative retinopathy is generally absent below 5 years' duration of diabetes and present in about 25% at 15 years and in over 50% at 20 years of diabetes. In older-onset diabetic patients, retinopathy can

Table 17.1. Appearances of diabetic retinopathy on fundoscopy and corresponding features on fluorescein angiography.

Stage	Features on fundoscopy	Angiographic appearances
Non-proliferative (background)	Featureless retina	Capillary dilatation Capillary occlusion (with areas of non-perfusion)
	Venous dilatation (generalized)	Confirmed
	Microaneurysms	Greater number visualized than by fundoscopy
	Haemorrhages*: • flame (superficial) • blot (deep in retina)	Haemorrhages appear as dark areas (fluorescence absorbed by haemorrhage)
	Exudates ('hard')	
Preproliferative	Cotton-wool spots**	Non-perfused areas, usually larger than cotton-wool spots and surrounded by dilated, leaky vessels
	Specific venous abnormalities: • loops • beading • reduplication	Appearances confirmed
	Arterial abnormalities: • segmental narrowing • 'sheathing' • occlusion	Reduced luminal size, irregularity
Proliferative	New vessels (neovascularization): • on disc • elsewhere (in periphery)	Abnormal configuration of leaky vessels
	Fibrous tissue	
	Advanced complications: Haemorrhage • preretinal • vitreous	
	Retinal detachment	Diffuse leakage

* A single retinal haemorrhage, in the absence of other features, is not diagnostic of diabetic retinopathy.
** A single cotton-wool spot, in the absence of other features, is not diagnostic of preproliferative retinopathy.

be present in the first few years of diabetes (about 3–4% for proliferative retinopathy) but the prevalence is lower than in young-onset diabetic patients after 15 or more years (about 15–20%).
• Macular oedema is also associated with increasing duration of diabetes. It is commoner in older-onset diabetic patients, particularly in the first few years after diagnosis.
• In younger-onset patients, the incidence of proliferative retinopathy is close to zero with less than 5 years' duration of disease. The 4-year incidence of proliferative retinopathy rises to 28% after 13–14 years of diabetes and is stable at 14–16% after 15 years.

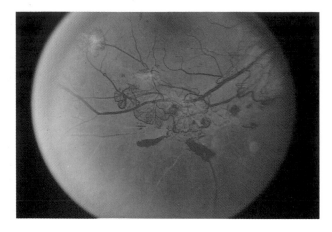

Fig. 17.5. New vessels arising elsewhere in the periphery of the retina (NVE), in this case inferior to the macula. The picture also shows arteriolar obliteration and retinal ischaemia; the columns of blood are attenuated and some occluded arterioles are reduced to whitish lines (e.g. between the two haemorrhages lying below the new vessels).

• In older-onset patients, the 4-year incidence of proliferative retinopathy is 2–3%, even in those with disease of short duration (2 years or less).

Detection and management

• Full ophthalmological examination should be carried out at the time of diagnosis and at least annually thereafter in patients diagnosed after 30

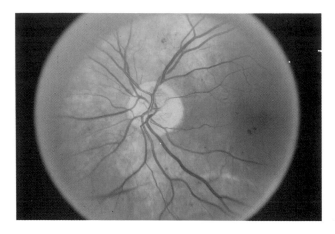

Fig. 17.6. Diabetic Retinopathy Study (DRS) standard photograph indicating new vessels on the disc, and showing a preretinal haemorrhage (at 7 o'clock).

years of age. In those diagnosed diabetic before this age, examination should be performed at least annually after 5 years of diabetes (Table 17.2).
• Ophthalmological referral is indicated soon for preproliferative changes; urgently for maculopathy, new vessel formation or retinal detachment; and immediately for vitreous haemorrhage or neovascular glaucoma (Table 17.3).
• It is now possible to treat the major sight-threatening complications of diabetic retinopathy (proliferative changes and macular oedema) using laser photocoagulation (Table 17.4, Fig. 17.11).
• Photocoagulation employs either the xenon arc

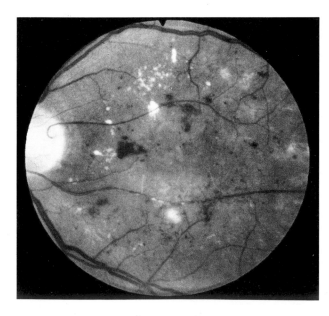

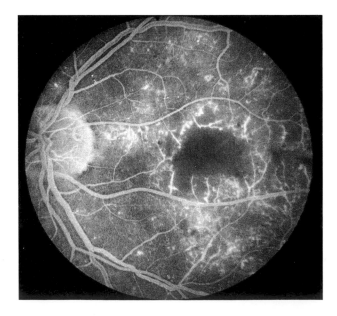

Fig. 17.7. (a) Right macular region of patient with ischaemic maculopathy. Note large blot haemorrhages suggesting ischaemia. (b) Fluorescein angiogram of area shown in (a). Note large perifoveal and peripheral ischaemic areas.

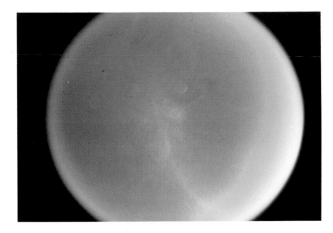

Fig. 17.8. Shows severe vitreous haemorrhage. The fundus is virtually invisible.

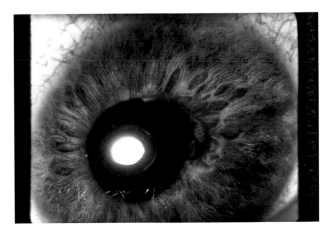

Fig. 17.9. Rubeosis iridis, most easily seen at 6 o'clock on the pupil margin. There is also circumcorneal injection of the sclera.

Fig. 17.10. Frequency of retinopathy (any degree) or proliferative retinopathy by duration of diabetes in persons taking insulin who were diagnosed as diabetic before 30 years of age who participated in the Wisconsin Epidemiologic Study of Diabetic Retinopathy, 1980–2.

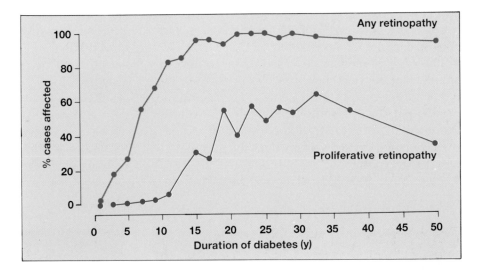

Table 17.2. Examination of the eyes in diabetic patients.

When to examine:
- On diagnosis
- Annually after 5 years of diabetes or if aged >30 years at diagnosis
- Annually if background retinopathy alone is present
- Three- to 6-monthly if retinopathy is more severe than background
- Immediately if any change in vision or visual symptoms occur

Examination should include:
- Visual acuity — distant vision (Snellen chart + spectacles or pinhole)
  — near vision (reading chart)
- Afferent pupillary defect
- Ophthalmoscopy through dilated pupils (1% tropicamide), unless glaucoma or previous eye surgery are present: examine lens, vitreous and retina

Specialized ophthalmological examination will also include slit-lamp microscopic examination of the iris, anterior chamber and retina, indirect binocular fundoscopy and measurement of intra-ocular pressure.

Condition	Urgency
Cataract	Routine (few months)
Hard exudates: close to macula or numbers increasing Retinal haemorrhages: numbers increasing Preproliferative changes	Soon (few weeks)
Fall in visual acuity (two lines or more) Visible maculopathy (oedema, exudates) New vessels Rubeosis iridis Advanced diabetic eye disease, especially retinal detachment	Urgent (1 week)
Vitreous haemorrhage Neovascular glaucoma	Immediate (same or next day)

Table 17.3. Indications for referring a diabetic patient to an ophthalmologist.

lamp, which produces a relatively large, painful retinal burn, or the argon laser, which has a smaller spot size.

• Photocoagulation can be used either to destroy specific targets (e.g. new vessels) or to treat the whole retina except for the central macula and the maculo-papillary bundle essential for central vision; this pan-retinal photocoagulation reduces overall retinal ischaemia and thus the stimulus to new vessel formation.

• Pan-retinal photocoagulation reduces by over 50% the likelihood of severe visual loss (acuity 1/60 or worse) developing in eyes with high-risk proliferative retinopathy. The place of photocoagulation in *preproliferative* changes is not yet established.

• Photocoagulation to the peripheral macula can also seal points of capillary leakage and so reduce macular oedema; photocoagulation treatment of clinically significant macular oedema (i.e. involving or threatening the fovea) reduces the risk of visual loss by over 50%.

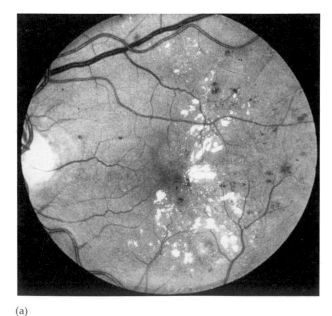

(a)

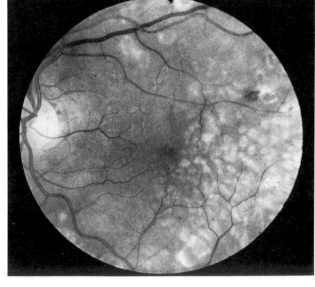

(b)

Fig. 17.11. (a) Hard exudate ring near the left macula, before treatment. Visual acuity 6/18. (b) Hard exudate ring has disappeared after treatment by pan-retinal photocoagulation. Visual acuity 6/9.

Table 17.4. Proliferative and preproliferative diabetic retinopathy. Indications for laser photocoagulation.

Condition	Recommended action
NVD	Pan-retinal photocoagulation before vitreous haemorrhage occurs
NVE	Pan-retinal photocoagulation before retinal detachment occurs
Rubeosis iridis	Pan-retinal photocoagulation before neovascular glaucoma develops
Preproliferative	Pan-retinal photocoagulation, of first eye
Peroperative	Pan-retinal endolaser photo-coagulation of all attached retina

NVD: new vessels on the disc; NVE: new vessels elsewhere.

Table 17.5. Useful services and facilities available in some countries for partially sighted and blind patients. Details in parentheses indicate UK availability.

Talking books. Giant cassette tapes and the machines for playing them (available from RNIB, British Talking Book Service for the Blind, Royal National Library for the Blind and Calibre Library)

Talking newspapers. Some papers and monthly magazines are available on standard cassettes (from the Talking Newspaper Association; some local authorities also provide local papers on cassette)

Library services. Most libraries have large-print books and some have a service for housebound readers

Residential establishments, courses, holiday homes and caravans for the blind (organized by the RNIB)

Information and a wide range of aids to daily life are available from blind associations (from the RNIB and the Partially Sighted Society)

RNIB=Royal National Institute for the Blind.

● Closed vitreo-retinal surgery is performed using instruments and a light source inserted into the vitreous cavity through the pars plana to avoid damaging the lens or retina. The eye is kept distended by a saline infusion. Fibrous membranes, haemorrhages and vitreous can be removed and

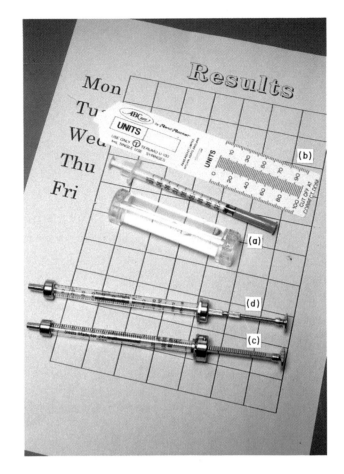

Fig. 17.12. A selection of aids for the blind and partially sighted: a large-print result sheet, magnifier and syringe guide, click count syringe and pre-set syringe.

detached areas of retina can be re-attached.

● Detached retina only remains viable for some weeks; detachment must therefore be diagnosed immediately if surgical re-attachment is to restore vision. B-scan ultrasonography can identify retinal detachments behind dense vitreous haemorrhages.

● Vitreo-retinal surgery can restore and maintain useful vision in up to 70% of eyes with advanced diabetic disease.

● Many aids are available to help blind and partially sighted patients to draw up insulin accurately and measure their blood glucose concentration (Fig. 17.12).

● It is essential to register blind or partially sighted patients immediately to activate the many social services and facilities available to them (Table 17.5).

18: Diabetic neuropathy: epidemiology and pathogenesis

- Diabetic neuropathy can be classified as either reversible (e.g. reduced nerve conduction velocity) or established (focal, multifocal, symmetrical and mixed neuropathies) — see Table 18.1.
- The epidemiology of diabetic neuropathy is unclear because of inconsistent definitions of what constitutes neuropathy — frequencies of 10–100% of patients affected have been reported. About 10% of patients have clinical signs and a further 10% also have symptoms. The prevalence and incidence of neuropathy both increase with the duration of diabetes (Fig. 18.1). Neuropathy is rare at the presentation of IDDM but may be present when NIDDM is diagnosed. The median time from the diagnosis of NIDDM to the onset of neuropathy is 9 years.
- Nerve biopsies show axonal degeneration and regeneration, demyelination and remyelination, and abnormalities of the vasa nervorum; capillary closure is correlated with the severity of neuropathy.
- Neurophysiological studies show reduced motor and sensory nerve conduction velocities and resistance to the failure of conduction which normally occurs when the nerve is rendered ischaemic.
- The pathogenesis is uncertain: metabolic factors may predominate in early disease and vascular factors at a later stage and in focal neuropathies.
- In experimental diabetic neuropathy, a possible metabolic mechanism involves hyperglycaemia-induced sorbitol accumulation, myoinositol depletion, reduced Na^+-K^+-ATPase activity and an increase in intracellular Na^+ levels (Fig. 18.2).
- The importance of non-enzymatic glycosylation of axonal proteins and changes in axoplasmic transport is uncertain.
- Neuropathy may develop acutely during periods of poor glycaemic control and may also be precipitated by weight loss (Fig. 18.3). Symptoms often tend to resolve when glycaemic control is improved or weight regained.

Clinical aspects of diabetic somatic neuropathy

- Diabetic peripheral neuropathy may present as several syndromes which often overlap (Fig. 18.4).
- *Chronic insidious sensory neuropathy* causes progressive development of unpleasant sensations, often with pain and hyperaesthesia, in the legs and feet. Muscle wasting and autonomic dysfunction are commonly associated. This form is common and usually unrelated to glycaemic control.
- *Acute painful neuropathy* and *diabetic amyotrophy* both cause sudden-onset pain in legs and/or thighs, usually unilateral in amyotrophy, associated with severe muscle wasting (Fig. 18.5) and occasionally profound weight loss; there is little objective sensory loss. These often begin during a period of hyperglycaemia and may improve with strict control.
- *Diffuse motor neuropathy* presents as severe, generalized muscle wasting and weakness, usually without pain or sensory loss (Fig. 18.6). It commonly affects older NIDDM patients; recovery is usually poor.
- *Focal neuropathies* are probably due to *pressure damage* (especially the carpal tunnel syndrome, which usually responds poorly to surgical decompression) or *vascular damage* (e.g. third nerve palsy, which is often painful, sometimes associated

Table 18.1. A classification of diabetic neuropathy.

Rapidly reversible phenomena:
 Distal sensory symptoms
 Reduced nerve conduction velocity
 Resistance to ischaemic conduction failure

'Established' neuropathy:
 Focal and multifocal neuropathies
 - cranial mononeuropathies
 - thoracoabdominal neuropathy
 - focal limb neuropathies
 - asymmetric proximal lower limb motor neuropathy (diabetic amyotrophy)

 Symmetrical neuropathies
 - sensory/autonomic polyneuropathy
 - proximal lower limb motor neuropathy

 Mixed syndromes

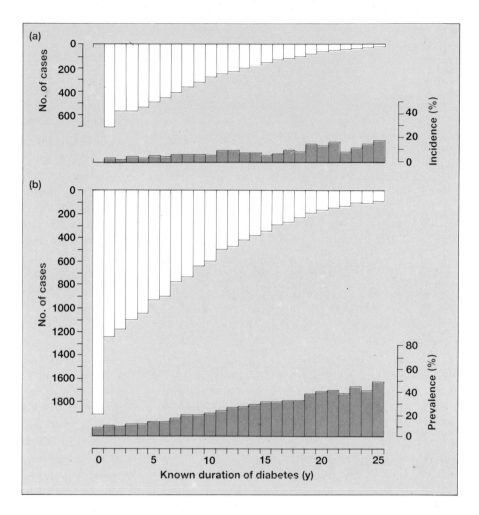

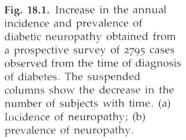

Fig. 18.1. Increase in the annual incidence and prevalence of diabetic neuropathy obtained from a prospective survey of 2795 cases observed from the time of diagnosis of diabetes. The suspended columns show the decrease in the number of subjects with time. (a) Incidence of neuropathy; (b) prevalence of neuropathy.

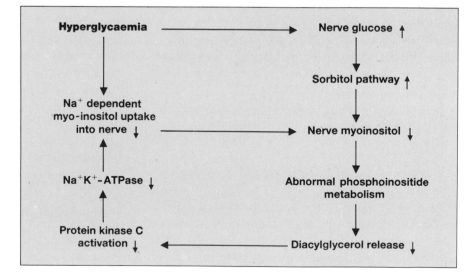

Fig. 18.2. Scheme summarizing proposed relationships between hyperglycaemia, sorbitol and myoinositol metabolism in peripheral nerve.

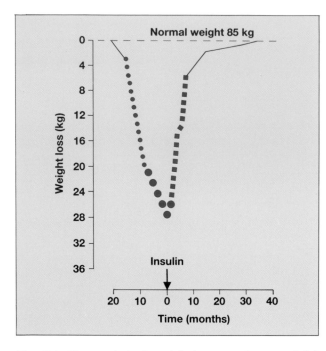

Fig. 18.3. Changes in body weight in a case of acute painful diabetic neuropathy. Initiation of treatment with insulin is indicated by the arrow, treatment before then having been with an oral hypoglycaemic agent. A precipitate loss of over 27 kg in weight is accompanied by the development of a mild (●) and then a severe (⬤) painful neuropathy. Restoration of body weight is associated with improvement (■) and then disappearance (———) of the neuropathy.

with hyperglycaemia and may recover with improved control — see Fig. 18.7).
● Other coexistent and potentially treatable causes of peripheral neuropathy (such as ethanol abuse or vitamin deficiency) must always be excluded.
● Leg pain in diabetic patients is also commonly due to vascular disease.

Assessment of peripheral nerves

● Peripheral nerve function can be assessed adequately by routine physical examination. Specialized tests for diagnostic difficulties and research applications include electrophysiological measurements of sensory and motor nerve conduction, determinations of vibration and thermal discrimination thresholds, and sural nerve biopsy (Table 18.2).

Management of diabetic isomatic neuropathy

● The main indication for intervention in neuropathy is pain and other troublesome sensory symptoms. A suggested management scheme is outlined in Fig. 18.8. Having excluded other possible causes and evaluated the extent of peripheral vascular disease, glycaemic control should first be improved as far as possible (e.g. by introducing or intensifying insulin treatment).
● Painful symptoms in diabetic neuropathy may respond to simple analgesia and tricyclic drugs (e.g. imipramine, often given together with fluphenazine at night); other agents (e.g. phenytoin, carbamazepine, mexiletine) are sometimes effective.

Autonomic neuropathy

● Up to 40% of diabetic patients show some evidence of autonomic dysfunction, but only a few have symptoms of autonomic neuropathy. As with peripheral diabetic neuropathy, autonomic nerve damage has been attributed to the metabolic consequences of hyperglycaemia. Both IDDM and NIDDM patients are affected.
● Autonomic neuropathy may evolve through defects in thermoregulation and sweating in the legs, followed by impotence and bladder dysfunction, to cardiovascular reflex abnormalities. Late manifestations include generalized sweating disorders, postural hypotension, gastrointestinal problems and reduced awareness of hypoglycaemia (Fig. 18.9).

Diagnosis of autonomic neuropathy

● Autonomic dysfunction is best diagnosed by evaluating the cardiovascular reflex responses to various stimuli. These stimuli include: changes in heart rate; to the Valsalva manoeuvre in response deep breathing and standing up; and blood pressure changes following standing and sustained hand-grip (see Table 18.3). These tests are simple, non-invasive and can be performed in the clinic within 30 minutes. Computer programs are available to analyse the results.

Syndrome	Chronic insidious sensory neuropathy	Acute painful neuropathy	Proximal motor myopathy	Diffuse motor neuropathy	Focal nerve palsies	
					Pressure (Median, Ulnar, Common peroneal)	'Vascular' (III, IV, VI; VII; Phrenic; Thoracic)
Pattern	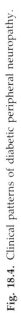					
Sensory loss	+→++	+	0	0→+	++	++
Pain	0→+++	+++	+→+++	0	++	0→++
Tendon reflexes	→	→	→	→	+	+
Muscle wasting and weakness	0→++	+→++	+++	++→+++	+→++	0→++
Autonomic features	+→++	May be present	May be present	May be present	May be present	May be present
Prevalence and relationship to glycaemia	Common; usually unrelated to glycaemia	Relatively rare; onset often during hyperglycaemia	Relatively rare; onset often during hyperglycaemia	Relatively rare; generally unrelated to hyperglycaemia	Relatively rare; usually unrelated to hyperglycaemia	Relatively rare; sometimes related to hyperglycaemia

Fig. 18.4. Clinical patterns of diabetic peripheral neuropathy.

Table 18.2. Assessment of peripheral nerve function.

Pathway		Modality	Clinical screen	Specialized tests	Comments
Sensory	Dorsal columns	Vibration	Tuning fork	Vibration perception threshold (VPT) measured with biothesiometer	Tuning fork unreliable; VPT varies with age and site and may be poorly reproducible
		Proprioception	Joint position, Romberg test	—	—
	Spino-thalamic	Light touch	Cotton wool	von Frey hairs	von Frey hairs are still a research procedure and not widely available
		Temperature	—	Thermal discrimination threshold (TDT), measured with Marstock thermode	May be more sensitive than VPT; time-consuming
	Single nerves	Pain	Pin-prick, deep pressure	Spring-loaded calipers to pinch skin; thermal pain threshold	Pain thresholds difficult to quantitate and poorly reproducible
			—	Electrophysiological measurements of sensory conduction velocity and action potential	Abnormalities early and common; include reduced conduction velocity and reduced amplitude with spreading of sensory action potential
Tendon reflexes			Ankles, knees (± reinforcement)	—	Ankle jerks often lost, but may be reduced or absent in elderly
Motor			Bulk, tone, power of limb muscles	—	Wasting of small hand muscles common in neuropathy, often with minimal weakness
			—	Electrophysiological measurements of motor conduction velocity	Motor nerve conduction velocity markedly reduced in clinical neuropathy, especially mixed forms

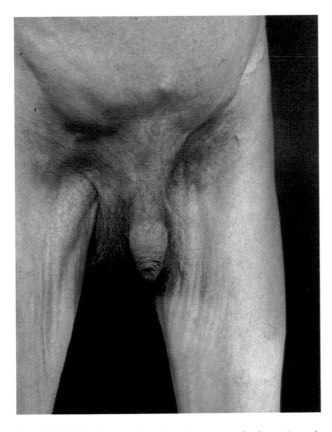

Fig. 18.5. Diabetic amyotrophy, showing marked wasting of both thighs.

- Other tests include measurements of pupillary function and sweating.
- The most prominent symptom is postural hypotension, which is due to loss of mainly sympathetic reflexes. It is aggravated by anti-hypertensive agents, antidepressants and insulin,

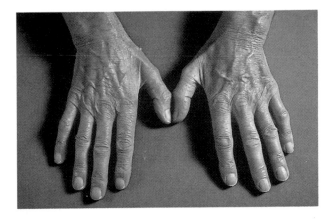

Fig. 18.6. Generalized wasting of small muscles of the hands due to diffuse motor neuropathy.

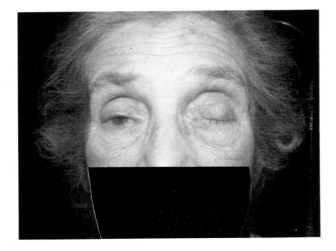

Fig. 18.7. Sudden onset of left ptosis (with diplopia) in a diabetic patient, due to third cranial nerve palsy. The patient complained of pain in the left orbit, and the left pupillary reactions were intact; pain and pupillary sparing are typical features of a third nerve palsy in diabetes.

Table 18.3. Normal, borderline and abnormal values for cardiovascular autonomic function tests.

	Normal	Borderline	Abnormal
Heart rate tests			
Heart rate response to Valsalva manoeuvre (ratio of longest to shortest R−R interval during, and after, manoeuvre)	≥1.21	—	≤1.20
Heart rate response to standing up (ratio of R−R interval at the 30th to the 15th heartbeat after standing up: the '30:15' ratio)	≥1.04	1.01−1.03	≤1.00
Heart rate response to deep breathing (maximum minus minimum heart rate)	≥15 beats/min	11−14 beats/min	≤10 beats/min
Blood pressure tests			
Blood pressure response to standing up (fall in systolic BP)	≤10 mmHg	11−29 mmHg	≥30 mmHg
Blood pressure response to sustained handgrip (increase in diastolic BP)	≥16 mmHg	11−15 mmHg	≤10 mmHg

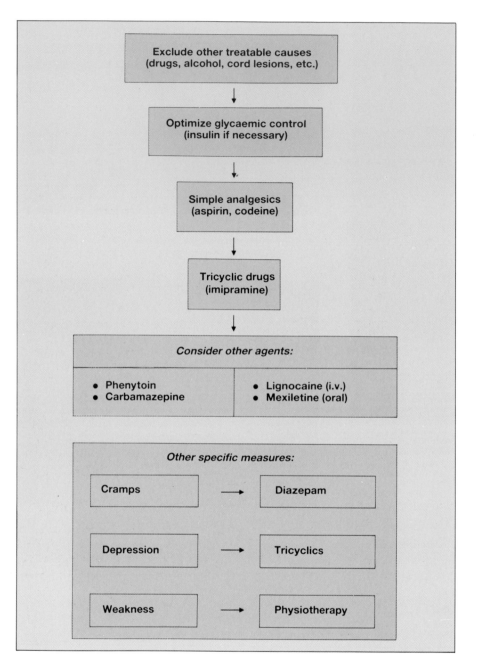

Fig. 18.8. Scheme of management of symptomatic diabetic neuropathy.

and may respond to fludrocortisone treatment.
• Bladder dysfunction usually causes asymptomatic enlargement but may cause overflow incontinence and recurrent urinary tract infections.
• Erectile failure is common in diabetic men, but is not always due to autonomic neuropathy.
• Symptomatic autonomic neuropathy carries a poor prognosis; death is usually due to associated diabetic complications (especially nephropathy) but is occasionally sudden and unexplained.

Management of autonomic neuropathy

• Neurogenic bladder problems may be helped by encouraging regular bladder emptying, if necessary by using manual suprapubic pressure every 3–4 h. Long-term single or cyclical chemotherapy may be indicated for recurrent or persistent urinary tract infections. Bladder neck

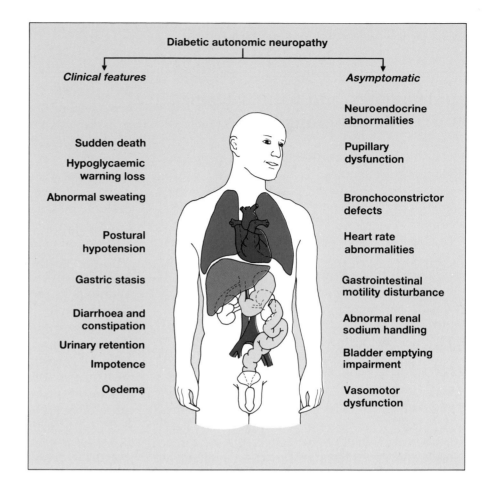

Fig. 18.9. Clinical features and asymptomatic effects of diabetic autonomic neuropathy.

resection may need to be considered in cases with large residual urine volumes, but may cause incontinence. Anticholinergic drugs may relieve sweating but may aggravate urinary retention.

• Postural hypotension only needs treatment if it is symptomatic. Mild symptoms during the day can be treated by raising the head of the bed a few centimetres at night. In those with more marked symptoms, fludrocortisone is the drug of choice. Glycaemic control may need to be relaxed in patients with impaired awareness of hypoglycaemia, which may coexist with autonomic neuropathy.

19: Diabetic nephropathy

Epidemiology and natural history of diabetic nephropathy

- Diabetic nephropathy is defined by persistent albuminuria (albumin excretion rate (AER) >300 mg/day; Albustix-positive), declining glomerular filtration rate (GFR) and rising blood pressure.
- Established nephropathy follows several years of incipient nephropathy, characterized by worsening microalbuminuria (AER, 30–300 mg/day) which is Albustix-negative and detectable by, for instance, radioimmunoassay. These stages are depicted in Fig. 19.1.
- The natural history of nephropathy differs between IDDM and NIDDM. In IDDM, nephropathy develops in about 35% of cases, especially in males and those whose diabetes presents before the age of 15 years. The incidence of nephropathy peaks after 15–16 years of diabetes and declines thereafter. In NIDDM, estimates of prevalence range from 3% to 16% and nephropathy often supervenes after a shorter known duration of diabetes than in IDDM.
- Nephropathy is rarer in NIDDM, but due to the relatively high prevalence of NIDDM, 50% of diabetic patients entering end-stage renal failure in Britain each year are non-insulin-dependent.
- The incidence of diabetic nephropathy is fall-ing, possibly due in part to improved diabetic management.
- In both IDDM and NIDDM, GFR begins to decline irreversibly when AER has risen to 100–300 mg/day, at an average rate of 10 ml/min/1.73 m^2 per year (Fig. 19.2). This is due to progressive reduction of the filtration surface area through mesangial expansion. Serum creatinine levels begin to rise when GFR falls below 50 ml/min/1.73 m^2 and end-stage renal failure follows after an average of 5 years.
- IDDM subjects with microalbuminuria have a 20-fold greater risk of ultimately developing clinical nephropathy than those with normal albumin excretion. Microalbuminuria also predicts clinical nephropathy and increased mortality in NIDDM. Nephropathic patients have an increased incidence of retinopathy and a ten-fold increase in cardiovascular mortality which is the major cause of death in nephropathic NIDDM patients.
- Other concomitants of albuminuria include increased urinary IgG excretion, hyperlipidaemia and elevated fibrinogen levels.

Aetiology and pathogenesis of diabetic nephropathy

- Albuminuria in diabetic nephropathy is due to glomerular capillary damage and reflects genera-

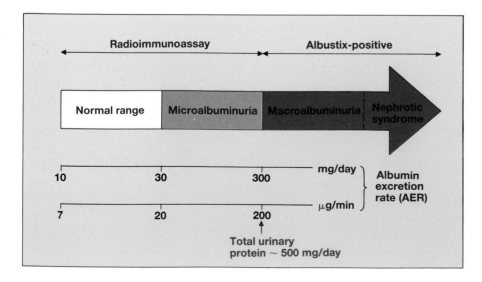

Fig. 19.1. Normo-, micro-, and macroalbuminuria.

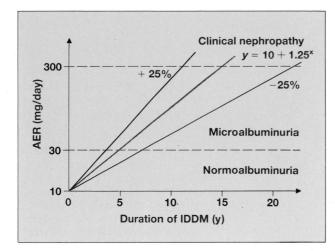

Fig. 19.2. Progression of microproteinuria and clinical nephropathy in IDDM, showing average rate and 25% confidence intervals for the increase in AER, plotted on a logarithmic scale.

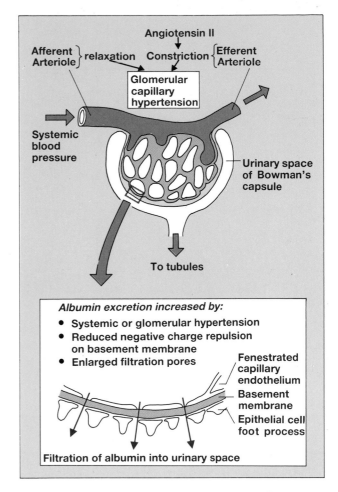

Fig. 19.3. Schematic diagram of glomerulus, indicating the main factors influencing excretion of albumin into the urine.

lized damage to the microcirculation and large vessels.

- Microalbuminuria is due to increased permeability of the glomerular capillaries, probably because of raised glomerular capillary pressure and loss of negative charge on the glomerular basement membrane. Clinical albuminuria develops with further loss of membrane charge and an increase in membrane pore size (Figs 19.3, 19.4).

- Non-diabetic renal disease accounts for proteinuria in up to 8% of diabetic patients. Alternative diagnoses are suggested by acute renal impairment, absence of retinopathy, haematuria, or short duration of IDDM (<5 years), and must be excluded by renal biopsy.

Hypertension and hyperfiltration

- Blood pressure is normal at the onset of IDDM and generally remains so in patients with normoalbuminuria. In microalbuminuric subjects, however, blood pressure begins to rise when AER exceeds 50 mg/day, although it often remains below the conventional threshold defining hypertension until clinical proteinuria supervenes.

- Hypertension accelerates the rates at which albuminuria increases and glomerular filtration rate declines. Conversely, the rate of progression of incipient and established nephropathy can be slowed and the associated mortality may be

reduced by aggressive antihypertensive treatment (Fig. 19.5).

- *Glomerular hyperfiltration* is an increase in glomerular filtration rate (GFR) above the normal range, which occurs early in 20–40% of IDDM patients. Possible causes of hyperfiltration include increased renal plasma flow and filtration surface area in the glomerulus.

- The glomeruli are hypertrophied and the kidneys enlarged. Hyperglycaemia and disturbances in the balance between vasodilating and vasoconstricting prostaglandins may contribute to hyperfiltration.

- The relationship of glomerular hyperfiltration (which does not apparently occur in NIDDM) to the subsequent development of clinical nephropathy is uncertain.

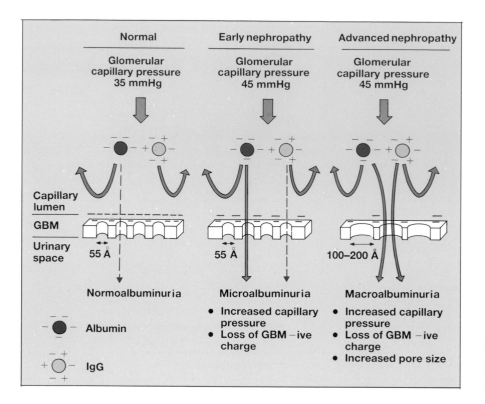

Fig. 19.4. The evolution of proteinuria in diabetes. Filtration of plasma proteins such as the polyanionic albumin and the larger electrically neutral IgG, is normally restricted by the resting negative charge on the glomerular basement membrane (GBM) and by the size of the filtration pores. Increased glomerular capillary pressure and loss of negative charge increase filtration of proteins, including albumin, in the early stage of microalbuminuria. With further loss of negative charge and enlargement of filtration pores in advanced nephropathy, albumin losses increase greatly and IgG is readily filtered.

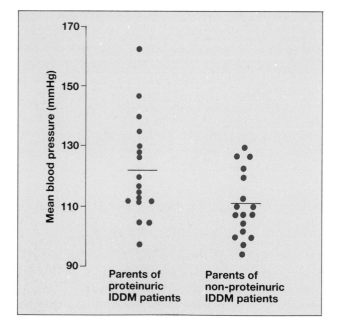

Fig. 19.5. Effect of antihypertensive treatment in reversing the steady increase in AER in an IDDM patient with microalbuminuria.

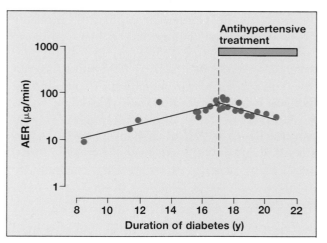

Fig. 19.6. Mean arterial blood pressure in the parents of proteinuric and non-proteinuric IDDM patients who were matched for age, sex and duration of diabetes.

Is there a genetic predisposition to nephropathy?

● The tendency to develop nephropathy may be partly genetically determined, as cases tend to cluster within families. A genetic predisposition to hypertension is suggested by the finding of increased blood pressure in the parents of diabetic patients with nephropathy (Fig. 19.6).

● Sodium/lithium countertransport activity in red blood cells (which reflects physiologically important cation exchange mechanisms) is increased in nephropathic patients and their parents; increased activity is a marker for essential hypertension. However, the consistency and significance of these findings has recently been questioned.

Structural changes in the diabetic kidney

- The characteristic histopathological features of the diabetic kidney occur in the glomerulus.
- The renal glomerulus comprises a tuft of 20—40 capillary loops arising from an afferent and drained by an efferent arteriole. The loops are arranged in lobules (Fig. 19.7) which are supported by mesangial tissue which has both cellular and acellular (matrix) components. Electron microscopy has shown that each loop is made up of a basement membrane lined by a fenestrated endothelium and covered by parietal epithelium. These epithelial cells are highly specialized podocytes which do not lie entirely on the basement membrane, but possess foot processes which interdigitate along the membrane, leaving small gaps (the filtration slits or pores) between them.
- Microalbuminuria is not always associated with structural abnormalities of the glomerulus.
- The major abnormalities are: increased glomerular volume secondary to basement membrane thickening and mesangial enlargement; hyaline deposits (of uncertain significance); and global glomerular sclerosis due to mesangial expansion or ischaemia, or both (Fig. 19.8).

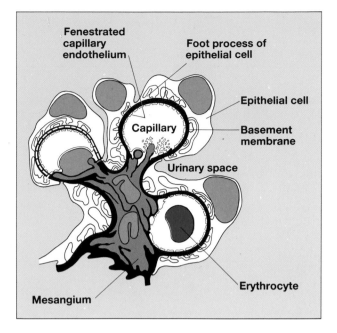

Fig. 19.7. Schematic representation of glomerular capillary tuft. Note continuity of glomerular basement membrane with mesangial matrix material (solid lines).

- Nodular accumulations of PAS-positive (*para*-aminosalicylic acid-positive) matrix material (the Kimmelstiel—Wilson lesion) are almost pathogenic of diabetic nephropathy (Fig. 19.9).
- GFR is closely correlated with the surface area of the glomerular capillary basement membrane (the filtration surface), itself determined by the number of glomeruli at diagnosis, the extent of

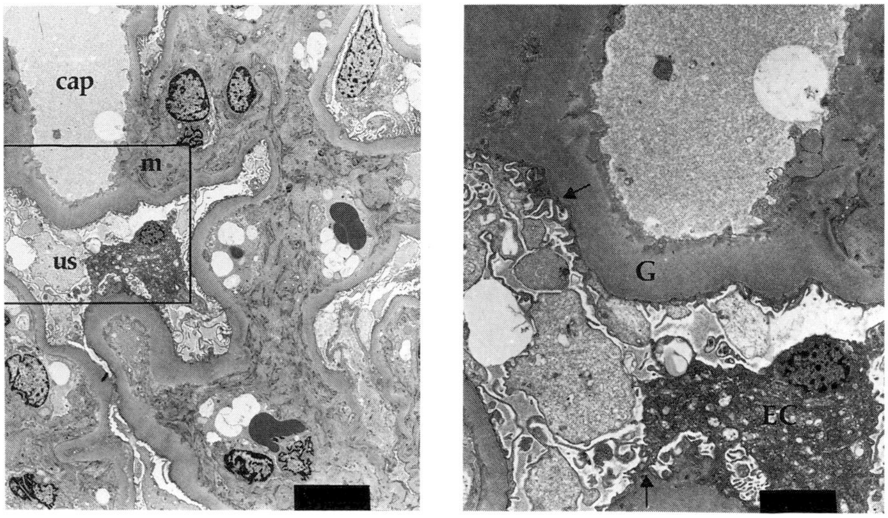

Fig. 19.8. Photomicrographs showing glomerular basement membrane thickening and mesangial expansion in the kidney of a diabetic patient. (a) ×1700; m = mesangial cell and matrix; us = urinary space; cap = capillary lumen. (b) ×4300, enlargement of boxed area in (a). G = glomerular basement membrane; EC = epithelial cell. Foot processes can be clearly seen (arrow).

(a)

(b)

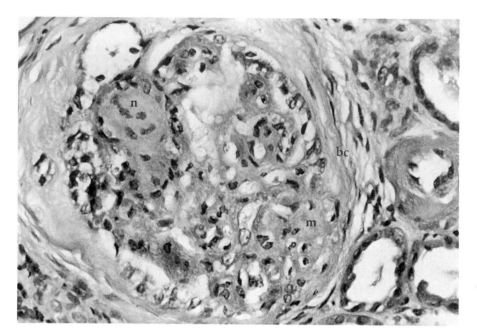

Fig. 19.9. Nodular glomerulosclerosis in a patient with diabetic nephropathy. Note thickened and split Bowman's capsule (bc) and obvious nodule (n). There is also diffuse mesangial expansion (m) (×600).

mesangial expansion, the capacity for expansion and the number of sclerosed glomeruli.

Clinical features of established diabetic nephropathy

• Patients with diabetic nephropathy may remain relatively asymptomatic until late in the natural history of the complication. The widespread introduction of screening for microalbuminuria has revealed many patients at earlier stages of nephropathy.

• Extensive, severe cardiovascular disease develops early in diabetic patients with nephropathy. Coronary heart disease is often asymptomatic but electrocardiographic and angiographic abnormalities are common. Peripheral vascular disease includes widespread multisegmental atheromatous lesions and medial arterial calcification in hands and feet; digital ischaemia and gangrene are common (Figs 19.10, 19.11). Virtually all patients with diabetic nephropathy are hypertensive.

• Neuropathic foot ulceration affects approximately one-quarter of diabetic patients with nephropathy, but Charcot joints are relatively uncommon. Tests of sensory and autonomic function are abnormal in most patients. Symptoms vary considerably.

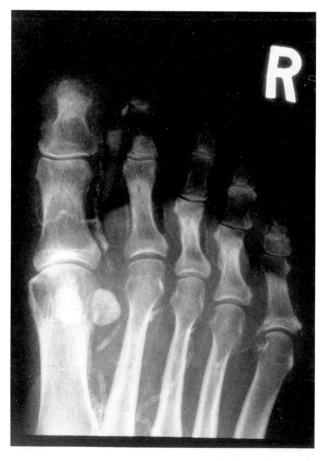

Fig. 19.10. Medial artery calcification in diabetic nephropathy.

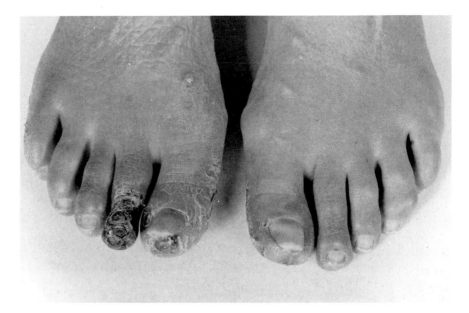

Fig. 19.11. Digital gangrene in diabetic nephropathy.

- The frequency of these other complications in diabetic patients with nephropathy is shown in Fig. 19.12.
- Retinopathy is virtually always present in nephropathy and is proliferative in about 70% of cases. Untreated retinopathy often deteriorates together with renal function, possibly through worsening hypertension and fluid retention.

Prognosis of diabetic nephropathy

- As is shown in Fig. 19.13 premature mortality is greatly increased at nearly all ages in proteinuric patients. Table 19.1 shows the causes of death in these patients.

Diagnosis and monitoring

- Non-diabetic causes of renal disease must be excluded.
- Once established, renal function in diabetic nephropathy tends to decline in a linear fashion, at a rate which is individual to the patient and may be determined by other factors, such as hypertension and smoking.
- Renal function must therefore be monitored in patients with diabetic nephropathy, both to estimate the time to end-stage renal failure and to determine the effects of intervention. Serum creatinine concentration does not reflect GFR in the early stages of nephropathy and only rises when

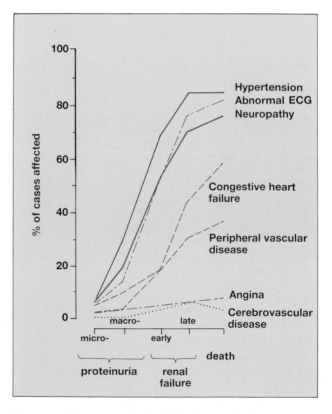

Fig. 19.12. Frequency of other diabetic complications at various stages of diabetic nephropathy.

GFR is reduced by 50–70% (Fig. 19.14). GFR should therefore be measured, ideally using isotopic methods, during the early stages. Serial plots of inverse creatinine (1000/creatinine in

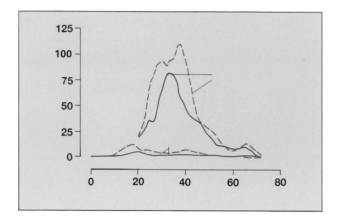

Fig. 19.13. Relative mortality of diabetic patients with and without persistent proteinuria, in men (——) and women (− −) as a function of age.

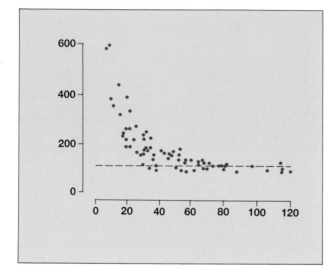

Fig. 19.14. Glomerular filtration rate (GFR) measured by ^{51}Cr-EDTA clearance, plotted against serum creatinine concentration in 73 subjects at various stages of diabetic nephropathy. Dashed line represents upper limit of normal serum creatinine concentration.

μmol/l) generally show a linear decline which, if extrapolated, may predict when end-stage renal failure is likely to occur (Fig. 19.15); this method is only useful when the serum creatinine concentration exceeds 200 μmol/l. The quantity of pro-

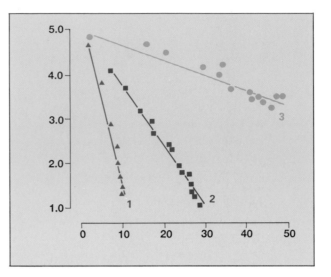

Fig. 19.15. Serial plots of inverse creatinine values (1000/serum creatinine concentration in μmol/l) in three representative diabetic nephropathic patients. Inverse serum creatinine declines linearly with time, at a fixed rate for each individual patient (fastest for patient 1 (▲) and slowest for patient 3 (●)).

teinuria and serum albumin levels should also be monitored.
● Urine must be cultured regularly to exclude infection, especially in patients with incomplete bladder emptying. Infection, dehydration and radiographic contrast media may precipitate acute-on-chronic renal failure.

Management of diabetic nephropathy

● This demands close cooperation between diabetic and renal physicians, and access to transplant surgeons and dialysis programmes. A general scheme is outlined in Fig. 19.16.
● In early diabetic nephropathy, treatment is largely preventative.
● Strict glycaemic control can reduce micro-albuminuria and lower glomerular hyperfiltration into the normal range. Effective antihypertensive

	UK study 1983	Steno	Joslin	UK study 1985
Renal failure	60%	66%	59%	50%
Cardiovascular disease	25%	24%	36%	25%

Table 19.1. Causes of death in diabetic nephropathy in two UK, one Danish (Steno) and a North American (Joslin) study.

Stage	Monitoring	Treatment

Microalbuminuria	• BP (3-monthly)
	• ? Echocardiography
	• Urinary albumin
	• Serum urea, creatinine and electrolytes
	• Glycaemic control
	• Serum lipids
		• Normalize BP
		• Optimize glycaemic control
		• Correct cardiovascular risk factors:
		  (a) dyslipidaemia
		  (b) smoking
		• Assess other diabetic complications and treat if possible

Macroalbuminuria as above, with:	• GFR (6–12-monthly); calculate interval to end-stage renal failure
	• Echocardiography (6-monthly)
	• ECG }
	• CXR } 12-monthly
	• Autonomic function tests
	• Somatic sensory tests
	• Regular fundoscopy (3–6-monthly)
	• Coronary and peripheral angiography if indicated
		• Consider low-protein diet
		• Regular review and treatment of diabetic complications:
		  (a) cardiac
		  (b) peripheral vascular
		  (c) feet (chiropodist)
		  (d) eyes

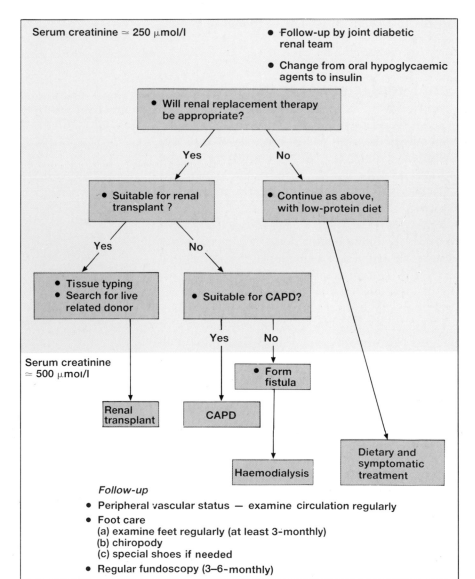

Fig. 19.16. Flow-chart illustrating the management of patients with diabetic nephropathy, before the onset of renal failure (upper panel), and with renal failure (lower panel).

treatment (Fig. 19.17) and restriction of dietary protein intake (to 45 g/day) can both reduce urinary albumin excretion. Angiotensin converting enzyme inhibitors may have an additional beneficial effect in reducing intraglomerular pressure. Whether these interventions influence the ultimate progression to clinical nephropathy is not known.

• Patients should be actively discouraged from smoking, which exacerbates vascular disease and may accelerate the progression of nephropathy.

Glycaemic control

• Insulin requirements fall (often by 50%) in renal failure due to reduced renal elimination of insulin. Metformin and most sulphonylureas are also cleared through the kidneys and accumulate in uraemia, causing hypoglycaemia and toxicity: transfer to insulin treatment is therefore recommended.

Renal replacement therapy

• Renal replacement therapy — renal transplantation, haemodialysis or continuous ambulatory peritoneal dialysis (CAPD) — should be offered as freely to diabetic as to non-diabetic patients as their survival rates are now nearly comparable (Fig. 19.18).

• Renal transplantation, ideally from a live related donor, is the treatment of choice in patients under 60 years of age. Transplantation is recommended when the serum creatinine reaches about 500 μmol/l. Five-year survival now exceeds 60% for cadaver grafts at most centres. Transplanted kidneys generally develop histological features of diabetic nephropathy but this is not known to have caused graft failure as yet.

• Chronic haemodialysis may be complicated in diabetic patients by difficult vascular access, postural hypotension and poor metabolic control and was previously associated with rapidly worsening retinopathy, causing blindness in 40% of cases. Haemodialysis may need to be started relatively early (serum creatinine 500−600 μmol/l) because of the tendency to fluid retention. Five-year survival is now about 45% and only 3% of cases now suffer visual loss; prognosis is poorer in patients over 60 years. Common causes of death are cardiovascular disease, sepsis and uraemia following withdrawal from dialysis.

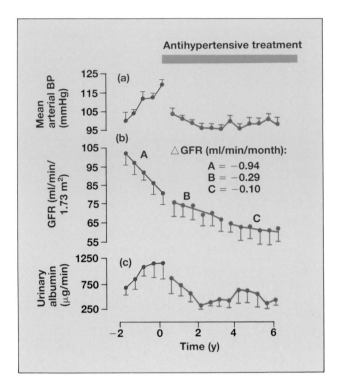

Fig. 19.17. Effects of antihypertensive treatment on mean arterial blood pressure (a), GFR (b) and urinary albumin excretion (c) in IDDM patients with nephropathy. Rate of decline in GFR and albumin excretion were both significantly reduced. Error bars are SEM.

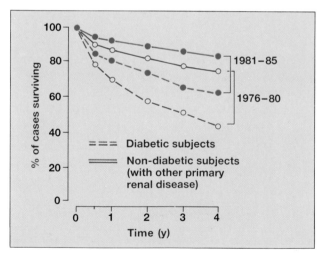

Fig. 19.18. Patient survival after first cadaver graft, for diabetic subjects and patients with other primary renal diseases, showing the improved survival of diabetic patients transplanted in 1981−85 (●) as compared with 1976−80 (○).

• CAPD is inexpensive, avoids rapid volume fluctuations and allows patients to be independent. It is suitable for elderly patients and those with ischaemic heart disease, severe autonomic neuropathy or visual impairment. Insulin (at about twice the usual subcutaneous dose) can be added directly to the dialysis fluid and is absorbed into the portal system. Peritonitis is no more common than in non-diabetic patients. Three-year survival is now about 60%.

• Coexistent vascular disease, retinopathy and foot problems must be identified and treated if possible before undertaking renal replacement therapy, and carefully monitored thereafter. Coronary heart disease is the major cause of death in the first few years after starting renal replacement therapy, accounting for 50–65% of deaths (10 times the rate in non-diabetic patients); patients receiving haemodialysis are particularly at risk. Strokes, digital and limb gangrene are also common.

20: Cardiac, macrovascular and hypertensive disease in diabetes

• Microvascular disease is an important cause of morbidity in diabetes, but diseases of the larger arteries and the heart are responsible for well over half of all deaths in diabetic patients. There is an association between micro- and macrovascular disease, as is demonstrated by the large excess of cardiovascular deaths in patients with proteinuria.

• Mortality from coronary heart disease (CHD) in diabetic patients is increased by about two and four times respectively for males and females, compared with the non-diabetic population.

• Deaths from cardiovascular disease predominate in patients with diabetes of over 30 years' duration, and in those diagnosed after 40 years of age.

• The frequency of CHD in diabetes is related to that in the background population (e.g. it is low in diabetic patients in China and Japan).

• General risk factors for cardiovascular disease include smoking, obesity, hyperlipidaemia, hypertension, insulin resistance, haemostatic and platelet abnormalities, lack of exercise and a positive family history. Specific diabetes-related risk factors may include hyperglycaemia (especially for peripheral vascular disease) and hyperinsulinaemia (Table 20.1).

Coronary heart and peripheral vascular disease in diabetes

• Coronary artery atherosclerosis may be more diffuse and severe than in non-diabetic subjects but the frequency of inoperable vessels is no higher, and the results and survival after coronary artery bypass grafting are now comparable with those in the general population. Coronary artery surgery or angioplasty should therefore be considered if medical treatment of angina is ineffective. The existence of a specific diabetic cardiomyopathy remains controverisal.

• Acute myocardial infarction in diabetes carries twice the mortality of that in the general population. Contributory factors may include coexistent diabetic cardiomyopathy, blunting of cardiac reflexes by autonomic neuropathy, and adverse cardiac and metabolic effects of increased non-esterified fatty acid levels.

• Acute myocardial infarction in diabetic patients should be managed with tight control of blood glucose and potassium levels and prompt treatment of cardiac failure; the role of thrombolytic drugs is not yet established and they should be avoided in proliferative retinopathy.

General	Diabetes-related
(a) Risk factors for coronary heart disease	
Smoking	Hyperglycaemia
Hypertension	Hyperinsulinaemia
Hyperlipidaemia	Proteinuria
Hypercoagulability	Microalbuminuria
Obesity	Both sexes affected equally
Lack of exercise	
Male sex	
Family history	
Oestrogen treatment	
(b) Approaches to risk reduction	
Stop smoking	
Optimize diabetic control	
Seek and treat hypertension	
Seek and treat hyperlipidaemia	
Give dietary advice	
• Optimizing diabetic control	
• Maintaining ideal body weight	
• Lowering lipid levels	
Encourage aerobic exercise	

Table 20.1. Risk factors for coronary heart disease and ways to reduce them.

• The symptoms of angina may be masked in diabetic patients by autonomic neuropathy.

• Angina may be treated by nitrates, calcium channel antagonists or β-blockers; other diabetic complications may influence the choice of drug.

• Breathlessness and exercise intolerance in a diabetic patient are often due to heart failure, in which physical examination and chest X-ray may be normal.

• Management of cardiac failure involves improved glycaemic control, treatment of hypertension and the use of nitrates, calcium channel antagonists, loop diuretics and angiotensin converting enzyme inhibitors.

• Half of all lower-limb amputations are performed in diabetic patients. However, proximal and distal bypass grafting now often achieve good results.

• All diabetic patients must be encouraged to stop smoking, as the premature mortality in diabetic smokers is about double that in the general population.

Lipoprotein abnormalities

The major lipoprotein classes can be separated by ultracentrifugation, and their characteristics and effects on atheroma are outlined in Table 20.2. Each comprises a hydrophobic core of triglycerides and cholesterol esters, surrounded by a coat containing polar phospholipids, free cholesterol and apoproteins. Their major metabolic pathways are outlined in Figs. 20.1, 20.2, 20.3.

• CHD in diabetic patients is associated with increased plasma cholesterol levels, with reduced high density lipoprotein-cholesterol (HDL-cholesterol) in NIDDM patients, and possibly with increased triglyceride levels.

• The most common lipid abnormality in diabetes is raised triglyceride levels due to excess very low density lipoprotein (VLDL) concentrations, caused by reduced clearance via the insulin-sensitive enzyme lipoprotein lipase and (in NIDDM) by increased VLDL production. Triglyceride levels often fall with intensified insulin treatment.

• Low density lipoprotein (LDL) levels are also increased in poor metabolic control, due to decreased clearance by LDL receptors which are stimulated by insulin and have a lower affinity for glycosylated apoprotein-B.

• HDL levels are reduced in NIDDM, in proportion to increased triglyceride and VLDL levels, but are relatively normal in IDDM; glycosylated HDL may be cleared more rapidly from the circulation.

• Hyperlipidaemia can be assessed from measurements of fasting plasma total cholesterol, HDL-cholesterol and triglyceride levels and calculation of LDL-cholesterol.

• Hyperlipidaemia is managed by improving metabolic control, dietary modification, stopping

Table 20.2. Lipoprotein classification.

	Chylomicrons	VLDL	IDL	LDL	HDL
Diameter (nm)	80–500	30–80	25–35	20	10
Electrophoresis	Origin	Pre-beta	Broad beta	Beta	Alpha
Principal core lipid	Exogenous triglyceride	Triglyceride Cholesterol esters	Cholesterol esters Triglyceride	Cholesterol esters Triglyceride	Cholesterol esters
Effect on atheroma	Nil	+	++	+++	Protects
Major apoproteins	AI and II B48 CII and III E	B100 CII and III E	B100 E	B100	AI and II CIII
Dietary and drug treatment for elevated levels	Diet Drugs ineffective	Fibrates Nicotinic acid ω-3 (N-3) fish oils HMG CoA reductase inhibitors	Fibrates Nicotinic acid	Resins Nicotinic acid Fibrates Probucol HMG CoA reductase inhibitors	Fibrates Nicotinic acid ω–3 (N-3) fish oils Resins raise HDL Probucol lowers HDL

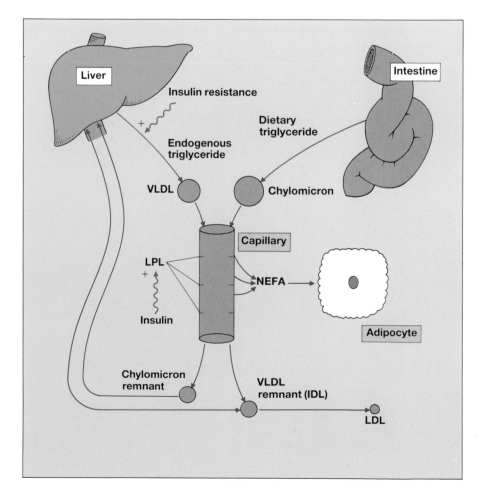

Fig. 20.1. Very low density lipoprotein (VLDL), containing endogenous triglyceride, and chylomicrons, containing dietary triglyceride, are catabolized by the endothelial enzyme lipoprotein lipase (LPL), releasing non-esterified fatty acids (NEFA) for use as fuel or storage in adipose tissue. The resulting remnant particles may be taken up by the liver, and the VLDL remnant (intermediate-density lipoprotein or IDL), containing all its original cholesterol, may be further catabolized to produce low density lipoprotein (LDL).

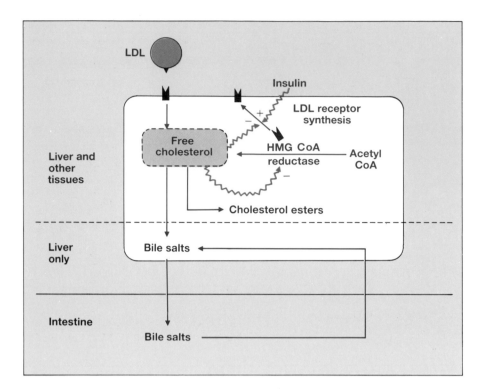

Fig. 20.2. Low density lipoprotein (LDL) is taken up predominantly via a receptor recognizing apoprotein B100. Free cholesterol is released into the cytoplasmic pool, which also receives endogenously synthesized cholesterol. The cholesterol is used in membrane and bile-salt synthesis or stored as cholesterol ester. The free cholesterol inhibits both LDL receptor synthesis and the activity of HMG CoA reductase, the rate-limiting enzyme in cholesterol synthesis, thus regulating its own concentration.

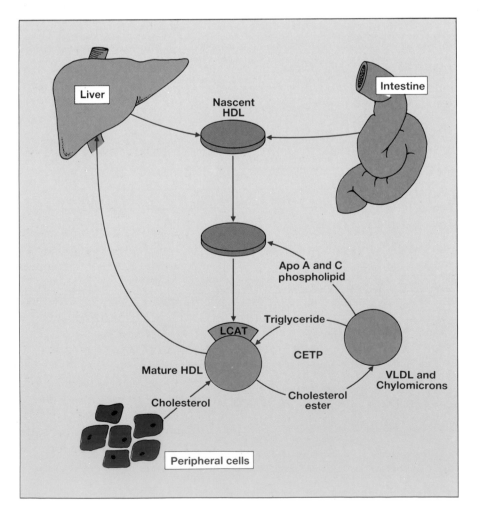

Fig. 20.3. High density lipoprotein (HDL) is produced as a lipid-poor disc. It receives apoproteins and phospholipids from triglyceride-rich lipoproteins, and the enzyme lecithin:cholesterol acyltransferase (LCAT) is activated by apo AI. It can then receive cholesterol from peripheral cells, esterify it and transport it to the liver either directly or by transferring it to other lipoproteins via cholesterol ester transfer protein (CETP).

Table 20.3. Guidelines for management of hyperlipidaemia. Adapted from the guidelines of the European Atherosclerosis Society.

Group	Lipid level (mmol/l)	Assessment	Treatment
A	Cholesterol 5.2–6.5 Triglyceride <2.3	Assess overall risk of CHD	Restrict food energy if overweight; give nutritional advice and correct other risk factors. If high risk, monitor as in B
B	Cholesterol 6.5–7.8 Triglyceride <2.3	Assess overall risk of CHD	Restrict food energy if overweight; prescribe lipid-lowering diet and monitor response and compliance. If cholesterol remains high, consider lipid-lowering drugs
C	Cholesterol <5.2 Triglyceride 2.3–5.6	Seek underlying cause	Restrict food energy if overweight; treat underlying causes if present. Prescribe and monitor lipid-lowering diet. Monitor response and compliance
D	Cholesterol 5.2–7.8 Triglyceride 2.3–5.6	Assess overall risk of CHD Seek underlying cause	Proceed as for group C above. If response is inadequate and overall CHD risk is high, consider lipid-lowering drugs
E	Cholesterol >7.8, or Triglyceride >5.6	Make full diagnosis	Consider referral to lipid clinic or specialized physician for investigation and treatment

smoking and specific lipid-lowering drugs (Table 20.3).

● A high-carbohydrate, low-fat (20–30% of total calories, 50% being unsaturated fat), low-cholesterol diet may lower cholesterol levels in IDDM. In NIDDM, weight reduction frequently lowers triglyceride concentrations and raises HDL (Table 20.4).

● Lipid-lowering drugs suitable for use in diabetes include the fibrates (bezafibrate, gemfibrozil) for hypertriglyceridaemia or mixed hyperlipidaemia, and the resins (e.g. cholestyramine) and HMG CoA reductase inhibitors ('statins', e.g. simvastatin, pravastatin) for hypercholesterolaemia.

● A suggested flow-chart for the management of hyperlipidaemia in diabetic patients is shown in Fig. 20.4.

Hypertension in diabetes mellitus

● Hypertension in diabetes represents an important health problem as the combination of the two diseases is common, carries significant morbidity and mortality, and is frequently difficult to treat.

● Hypertension affects over 30% of European diabetic patients and is twice as common as in the non-diabetic population.

● The prevalence and natural history of hypertension differ between IDDM and NIDDM, as shown in Fig. 20.5.

Table 20.4. American Heart Association lipid-lowering dietary phases.

Phase I	30% calories as fat; equal proportions of saturated, monounsaturated and polyunsaturated; under 300 mg cholesterol
Phase II	25% calories as fat; equal proportions of fatty acid types; 200–250 mg cholesterol
Phase III	20% calories as fat; equal proportions of fatty acid types; 100–150 mg cholesterol

● The presence of hypertension in diabetic patients increases mortality four- to five-fold, largely through coronary heart disease and stroke. Women and Afro-Caribbean patients are particularly at risk.

● Hypertension may also be an aetiological factor in diabetic nephropathy (to which it may determine susceptibility) and retinopathy.

● Diabetes may predispose to hypertension by promoting sodium retention, increasing vascular tone and by contributing to nephropathy (Fig. 20.6). Hypertension in NIDDM may, like the commonly associated hyperlipidaemia, be partly a consequence of insulin resistance and hyperinsulinaemia. Other possible associations are shown in Table 20.5.

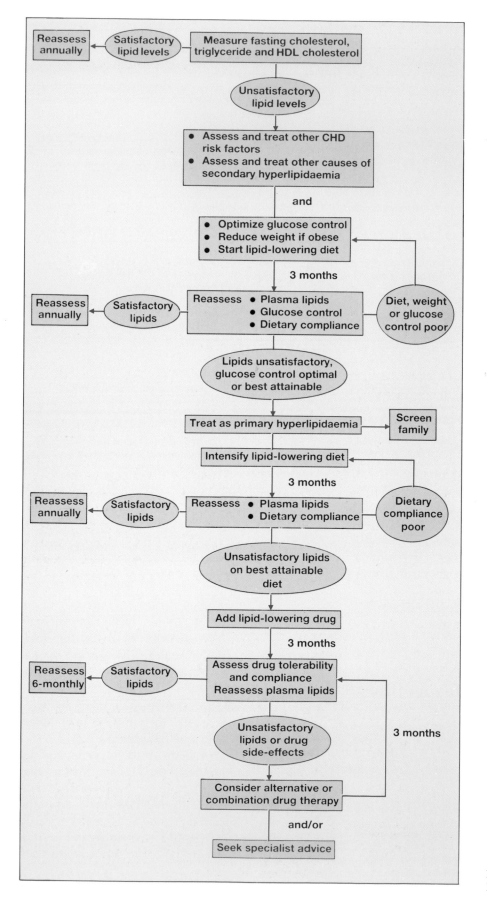

Fig. 20.4. Management of hyperlipidaemia.

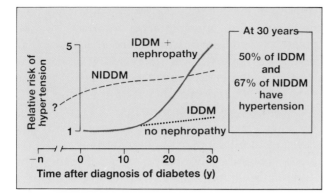

Fig. 20.5. Schematic time-course of development of hypertension in NIDDM patients, and in IDDM patients with and without nephropathy. The majority of hypertensive IDDM subjects are those with nephropathy.

Diagnosis and investigation of hypertension in diabetic patients

● All diabetic patients must have their blood pressure checked at diagnosis and at least annually thereafter. This is vitally important in patients with other cardiovascular risk factors, nephropathy (especially macroproteinuria, which is associated with a several-fold increase in cardiovascular mortality), or poor diabetic control.

● Blood pressure must be measured using an accurate sphygmomanometer and a cuff of an appropriate size (i.e. wider for NIDDM patients with fat arms). The WHO criteria in general use define hypertension as a blood pressure exceeding 160/95 and borderline hypertension as being

Table 20.5. Possible associations of diabetes with hypertension.

Endocrine diseases causing both hypertension and diabetes
Acromegaly
Cushing's syndrome
Conn's syndrome
Phaeochromocytoma

Drugs causing both hypertension and diabetes
Oral contraceptives (combined preparations)
Glucocorticoids

Antihypertensive drugs causing diabetes
Potassium-losing diuretics (especially chlorthalidone)
β-blockers
Diazoxide

Hypertension secondary to diabetic complications
Nephropathy
Renal scarring following recurrent urinary tract infections
Isolated systolic hypertension due to atherosclerosis

Hypertension associated with NIDDM, insulin resistance and hyperlipidaemia ('Syndrome X')

Hypertension associated with intensified insulin treatment

Coincidental hypertension in diabetic patients
Essential hypertension
Isolated systolic hypertension

below these limits but above 140/90 mmHg. Hypertension is diagnosed when readings consistently exceed 160/95 mmHg for several weeks, or when the pressure is very high (diastolic pressure >110 mmHg), or when there is clinical evidence of tissue damage due to long-standing hypertension. The WHO thresholds may be too

Fig. 20.6. Metabolic factors which may contribute to hypertension in diabetes. Sodium retention (due to both hyperglycaemia and high insulin levels) increases extracellular fluid (ECF) volume. Hyperinsulinaemia (in NIDDM, or during insulin treatment) also stimulates noradrenaline release, which together with enhanced vascular sensitivity to pressors, may increase peripheral resistance. Renin—angiotensin—aldosterone axis activity is generally suppressed by increased ECF volume and sodium load but is increased by volume depletion in ketoacidosis. Renin biosynthesis and release from the juxtaglomerular apparatus (JGA) may also be impaired in diabetes.

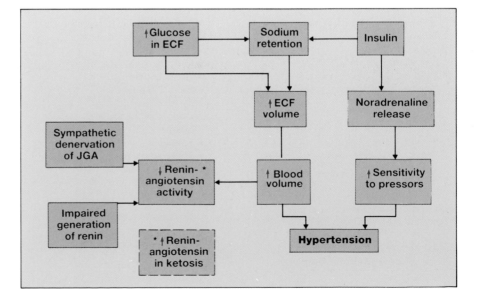

high in diabetic patients because of their additional risk of vascular disease.

• Initial investigations of the hypertensive diabetic patient must exclude rare causes of secondary hypertension, assess vascular and renal damage, and identify other cardiovascular risk factors.

• Secondary hypertension may be indicated by clinical findings of endocrine or renal disease, significant hypokalaemia (plasma potassium <3.5 mmol/l, without previous diuretic treatment), failure of hypertension to respond to standard treatment, or a sudden decline in renal function after starting treatment with ACE inhibitors (suggestive of renal artery stenosis). Baseline investigations are indicated in Table 20.6.

Management of hypertension in diabetes

• Treatment should lower blood pressure to a level where the additional morbidity and mortality attributable to hypertension are eliminated. This threshold in diabetic people is unknown, but while awaiting more precise information, and given the increased hazards of diabetes at all grades of hypertension, it seems reasonable to treat mild hypertension (>160/95 mmHg) in diabetic patients and probably to aim for the WHO target pressures (140/90 mmHg).

• General measures such as dietary advice and reducing alcohol intake may themselves normalize blood pressure. Education and stressing the importance of normalizing blood pressure in a non-threatening way, is also crucial to compliance. Other cardiovascular risk factors (particularly smoking and hyperlipidaemia) must be treated energetically.

• First-line antihypertensive drugs in diabetic patients include: diuretics at low dosage, to avoid adverse metabolic effects due to potassium depletion; cardioselective β-blockers, which may worsen metabolic control; calcium channel blockers, which do not affect metabolic control and have useful anti-anginal and antiarrhythmic effects; and ACE inhibitors, which have no metabolic side-effects and can reduce albumin excretion in diabetic nephropathy. Second-line drugs include vaso-

Table 20.6. Investigation of the diabetic patient with hypertension.

Physical tests	Questions to be answered
History Cardiovascular symptoms Previous urinary disease Smoking and alcohol use Medication Family history of hypertension or cardiovascular disease	*Is hypertension significant?* *Does hypertension have an underlying cause?* • Renal • Endocrine • Drug-induced

Examination
Blood pressure erect and supine
Left ventricular hypertrophy?
Cardiac failure?
Peripheral pulses (including renal bruits
  and radio-femoral delay)
Fundal changes
Evidence of underlying endocrine or renal
  disease
	Has hypertension caused tissue damage?
	• Left ventricular hypertrophy
	• Ischaemic heart disease
	• Cardiac failure
	• Peripheral vascular disease
	• Renal impairment
	• Fundal changes

ECG Left ventricular hypertrophy Ischaemic changes Rhythm	*Are other cardiovascular risk factors present?* • Smoking • Hyperlipidaemia • Poor glycaemic control • Positive family history
Chest radiograph Cardiac shadow size Left ventricular failure	
Blood tests Urea, creatinine, electrolytes Fasting lipids	

Table 20.7. Antihypertensive drugs used in diabetes.

Group	Examples	Dosage	Relative indications	Relative contraindications	Precautions
Diuretics	Bendrofluazide Hydrochlorothiazide Indapamide Frusemide	1.25–2.5 mg o.d. 25 mg o.d. 2.5–5 mg o.d. 40–80 mg o.d.	Cardiac failure Renal failure (frusemide)	Hyperosmolar coma Impotence Gout Hyperlipidaemia	Give with potassium supplements or ACE inhibitors Monitor blood potassium Check blood glucose and lipids
β-blockers (cardio-selective)	Atenolol Metoprolol	25–100 mg o.d. 50–100 mg b.d.	Angina Previous myocardial infarction	Cardiac failure Heart block Peripheral vascular disease Impotence Asthma, chronic airflow obstruction Hyperlipidaemia	Warn about loss of hypoglycaemic awareness Monitor blood glucose and lipids
ACE inhibitors	Captopril Enalapril	12.5–50 mg b.d. (6.25 mg initially) 10–40 mg o.d. (2.5–5 mg initially)	Cardiac failure Proteinuria	Renal artery stenosis Renal impairment	First-dose hypotension (use small starting dose at night) Monitor renal function Monitor plasma potassium (risk of hyperkalaemia)
Calcium entry blockers	Nifedipine Diltiazem Verapamil	20 mg b.d. (sustained release) 60–120 mg t.d.s. 120–240 mg b.d. (sustained release)	Angina Arrhythmias	Significant cardiac failure Treatment with digoxin + β-blocker (verapamil)	
Other agents	Labetolol Prazosin Hydralazine Clonidine	50–1200 mg b.d. 0.5–5 mg t.d.s. 25–50 mg b.d. 50–400 mg t.d.s.	Hypertensive crisis Impotence Renal failure Migraine		First-dose hypotension (prazosin) Use with diuretics and β-blockers

Dosage schedules: o.d., one daily; b.d., twice daily; t.d.s., thrice daily.

Combination	Specific benefits	Disadvantages
Diuretic + ACE inhibitor	ACE inhibitors prevent activation of angiotensin-aldosterone system due to diuretic-induced ECF volume contraction, and help to retain potassium	High risk of 'first-dose' hypotension with ACE-inhibitor in patients overtreated with diuretics
Diuretic + atenolol	—	Possibly aggravate hyperglycaemia in NIDDM
Diuretic + nifedipine	Diuretic reduces mild ankle swelling due to nifedipine	—
Atenolol + nifedipine	Atenolol counteracts tachycardia due to nifedipine's vasodilator action; effective anti-anginal therapy	May aggravate or provoke cardiac failure (both are negative inotropes)

Table 20.8. 'Logical' double-drug antihypertensive therapy.

Diuretics should be used in the lowest possible dose and combined with potassium supplements (or an ACE inhibitor) to minimize potassium depletion. Atenolol and nifedipine are used as examples of a β-blocker and a calcium channel blocker suitable for use in diabetic patients.

dilators and centrally acting agents (Table 20.7).
• Patients failing to respond to general measures should receive a single suitable first-line drug. Treatment failures should be given, in sequence: another suitable first-line drug; a logical combination of two first-line drugs (Table 20.8); and then triple therapy with another first-line drug or a vasodilator.
• Only 5% of patients will fail to respond to triple therapy; possible underlying causes of hypertension should be investigated and addition of a fourth drug (e.g. clonidine) may be helpful.
• Antihypertensive treatment is simply one aspect of a multipronged attack on cardiovascular risk factors. Any drugs must be chosen carefully to minimize any adverse effects on the patient's diabetic control, cardiovascular risks or quality of life. A treatment schedule is summarized in Fig. 20.7.

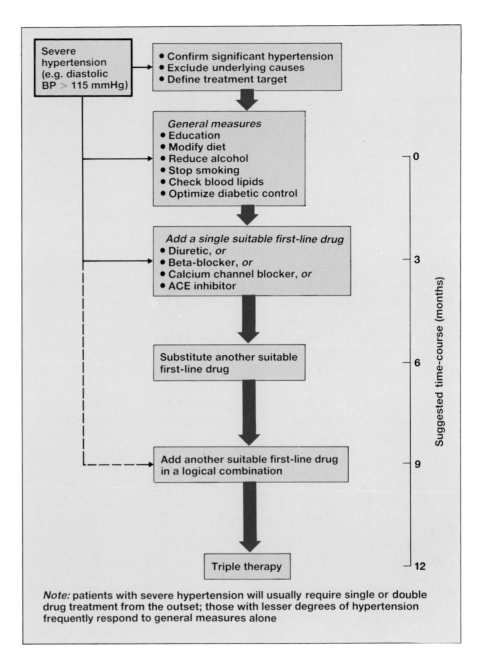

Fig. 20.7. Suggested management scheme for diabetic patients with hypertension. Drug treatment should be started as shown if hypertension remains uncontrolled after 3 months of general measures. Patients with severe hypertension will generally need drug treatment from the outset.

21: The diabetic foot

- Foot problems in diabetic patients are a common cause of chronic and expensive disability. Most of these problems can be prevented by effective education and screening of patients at risk.
- Both neuropathy and ischaemia, frequently acting in combination and often complicated by infection, predispose to ulceration in the diabetic foot.
- The neuropathic foot is numb, warm and dry, with palpable pulses; complications include neuropathic ulcers (Fig. 21.1), Charcot arthropathy and (rarely) neuropathic oedema.
- Neuropathic ulcers occur at points of high pressure loading, especially on the soles or at sites of deformity; pressure damage leads progressively to callosity formation, autolysis and finally ulceration (Fig. 21.2). Secondary infection is common. Treatment involves removing skin callosities to drain the ulcer, reducing pressure loading by special shoes or total-contact plaster casting (Fig. 21.3), and appropriate antibiotics.
- Charcot arthropathy usually involves the metatarso-tarsal joints, frequently follows minor trauma, and presents as warmth, swelling and redness, sometimes with pain (Fig. 21.4). Bone scans allow early diagnosis and radiographs later show dis-

organization of the joint and new bone formation (Fig. 21.5). Treatment is by immobilizing and unloading the limb, with non-steroidal anti-inflammatory drugs for pain.
- Neuropathic oedema may be due to micro-circulatory disturbances following autonomic denervation; ephedrine treatment is often effective.
- The ischaemic foot is cold and pulseless and subject to rest pain, ulceration and gangrene.
- Ischaemic ulceration usually affects the foot margins (Fig. 21.6). Medical treatment alone is often effective; focal stenoses of the iliac, femoral or even popliteal arteries are often amenable to angioplasty or bypass grafting; amputation must be avoided if at all possible, and limited ray excisions may prove satisfactory (Fig. 21.7).
- Infection is common in diabetic foot ulcers and often involves anaerobic organisms in addition to *Staphylococcus, Streptococcus* and other species such as *Proteus* and *Pseudomonas*. Gas formation (Fig. 21.8) and osteomyelitis are not uncommon sequelae. Long-term, intensive systemic antibiotic treatment may be needed (Table 21.1). The presence of cellulitis is an important warning sign which must be taken seriously.

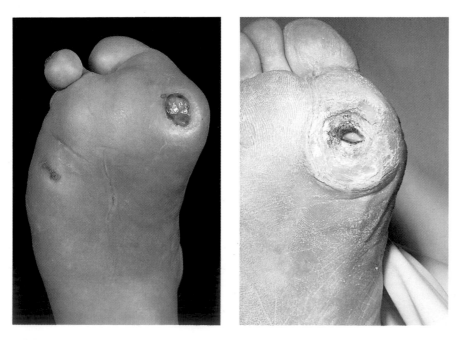

Fig. 21.1. Typical 'punched-out' neuropathic ulcers arising in heavily calloused skin underlying the first metatarsal head. Note previous amputations (left) and particularly thick callosities (right).

• The management of diabetic foot ulceration is best guided by determining the relative contributions of neuropathy, ischaemia and infection.

Collaborative teamwork involving the chiropodist, orthotist (shoe fitter), nurse, physician and surgeon is most effective.

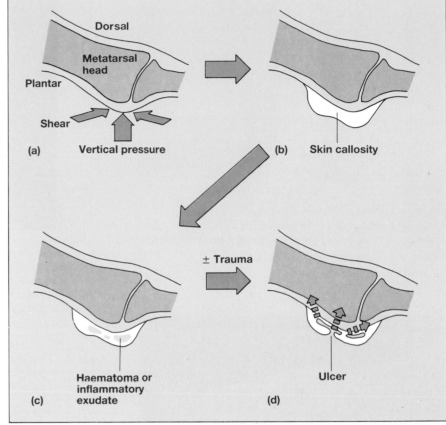

Fig. 21.2. Formation of a neuropathic pressure ulcer. (a) Abnormal foot posture and loss of sensation, both due to neuropathy, increase vertical pressure and tangential shear forces applied to vulnerable areas such as the metatarsal heads. (b) Increased pressure and shear forces cause hyperkeratosis and ultimately callosity formation. (c) Haematomas and inflammatory exudate (initially sterile) form within the callosity, finally breaking through to the surface to form an ulcer. (d) Trauma accelerates the process. Secondary infection may spread to cause soft-tissue necrosis or osteomyelitis.

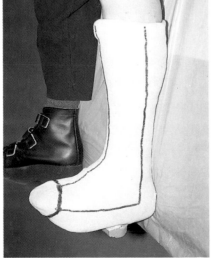

Fig. 21.3. Total-contact plaster cast used to treat neuropathic ulceration. Weight is taken by the plastic rocker, off-loading pressure from the ulcerated area. Lines show where the cast is cut for removal.

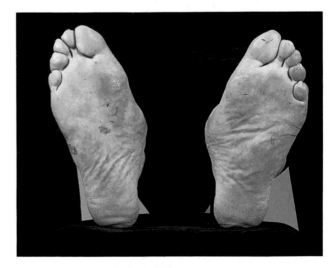

Fig. 21.4. Advanced Charcot arthropathy of both feet, showing gross disorganization. (Reproduced by kind permission of Dr Ian Casson, Broadgreen Hospital, Liverpool.)

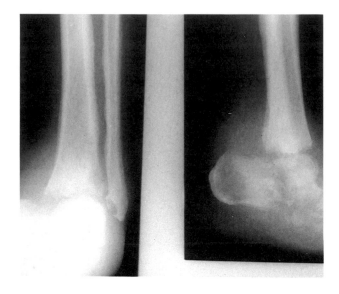

Fig. 21.5. Radiograph of advanced Charcot arthropathy, showing destruction of the ankle and foot joints, with widespread bone resorption, soft tissue swelling and a large effusion.

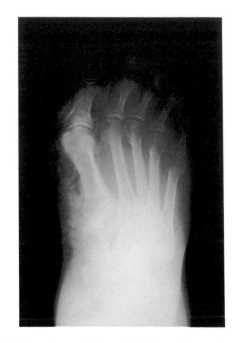

Fig. 21.8. Extensive soft-tissue infection with gas formation arising from a neuropathic ulcer in a diabetic foot. (Reproduced by kind permission of Dr Ian MacFarlane, Walton Hospital, Liverpool.)

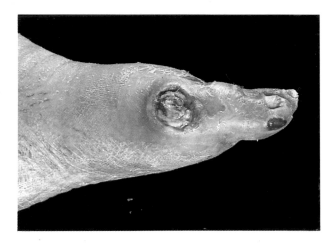

Fig. 21.6. Ulceration over the medial margin of the first metatarsal head in a neuro-ischaemic foot.

Table 21.1. Treatment of sepsis in the neuropathic foot.

- Admit to hospital
- Bedrest
- Antibiotics: 'general cover' regimen or specific, if organisms known:
  cefuroxime 1.5 g 8-hourly i.v. ⎫
  flucloxacillin 500 mg 6-hourly i.v. ⎬ 'general cover' regimen
  metronidazole 1 g 8-hourly rectally ⎭
- Urgent surgical drainage of pus and debridement of dead tissue
- Send pus and tissue for culture; adjust antibiotics accordingly
- Consider ray amputation of digit if bone is destroyed
- Ensure tight glycaemic control, using i.v. insulin if necessary

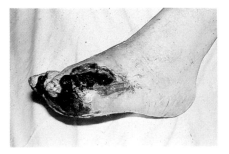

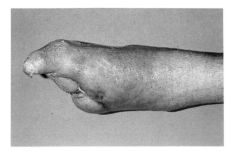

(a) (b)

Fig. 21.7. Distal gangrene in a neuro-ischaemic foot (a). After ray excision (b), the great toe is preserved and the foot remains able to maintain balance and walking.

Structured examination of the diabetic foot

• A scheme for the logical examination of the foot in a diabetic patient is shown in Table 21.2. The main aims are to determine the factors contributing to ulceration in an already affected foot, and to identify risk factors for future ulceration. Prevention is undoubtedly better than cure; patients' feet must be inspected regularly and they must be carefully educated to avoid factors predisposing them to damage (e.g. tightly or incorrectly fitting shoes) and to report the first signs of damage.

Table 21.2. Examination of the foot in a diabetic patient.

Colour:
• Red foot (cellulitis or early Charcot arthropathy)
• Pale or cyanotic foot (ischaemia)
• Pink foot associated with pain and absent pulses (severe ischaemia)

Deformity:
• Claw toe, hammer toe, hallux valgus, hallux varus
• Pes cavus, prominent metatarsal heads
• Charcot arthropathy

Oedema:
• Bilateral may be due to cardiac failure, fluid overload or neuropathy
• Unilateral may indicate sepsis or Charcot arthropathy

Nails:
• Atrophic in neuropathy and ischaemia
• Discoloured in fungal infection and subungual ulceration

Skin callosities:
• In the neuropathic foot, found on the plantar surface of the metatarsal heads and apices of toes

Tissue breakdown: ulcers
• Neuropathic typically on soles
• Neuro-ischaemic typically on foot margins

Tissue breakdown: fissures, blisters

Foot pulses:
• Posterior tibial and dorsalis pedis are weak or absent in ischaemic feet, often strong in neuropathic feet

Skin temperature:
• Neuropathic feet are usually warm, ischaemic feet are cold

Skin moisture:
• Neuropathic feet are dry

Signs of infection:
• Crepitus, fluctuation, deep tenderness

22: The skin in diabetes mellitus

• Skin disorders affect about 30% of diabetic patients. These conditions fall into four general categories (Table 22.1). This chapter will concentrate principally on disorders regarded as cutaneous markers of diabetes and the dermatological complications of treatment.

• Various skin conditions occur frequently in diabetes, although it now seems likely that several conditions previously regarded as cutaneous markers of diabetes (Table 22.1) are simply associated by chance. These conditions include necrobiosis lipoidica diabeticorum (NLD), granuloma annulare and diabetic dermopathy. Generalized pruritis has long been assumed to be associated with diabetes but this link also now appears to be spurious.

• Necrobiosis lipoidica diabeticorum (Fig. 22.1) consists of non-scaling plaques with atrophic epidermis and thick, degenerating collagen in the dermis, usually in the pretibial region. Surface telangiectases and a reddish border (sometimes raised) are characteristic.

• The histological hallmark of the condition (necrobiosis) refers to degeneration and thickening of collagen bundles in the dermis.

• Evaluation of NLD treatment, which must take into account the 20% spontaneous remission rate, has not yet been rigorously undertaken. Active red lesion margins may respond to steroids, either injected or applied locally, but topical steroids are contraindicated once atrophy is apparent; local emollients may then be used instead. Skin grafts of necrobiotic ulcers or lesions are often complicated by recurrence within or around the grafts.

• Granuloma annulare is an annular or arciform lesion with a raised papular border and flat centre, usually found on the dorsum of the hands and arms (Fig. 22.2). Histologically, there is mid-dermal collagen degeneration and abundant mucin. Rare generalized and perforating varieties have been described. No treatment is usually required. Diabetic dermopathy consists of bilateral pigmented pretibial patches (shin spots) which mostly affect older male diabetic patients. It is not strongly associated with diabetes, having been reported in 1.5% of healthy medical students. The typical appearance is shown in Fig. 22.3.

Table 22.1. The skin and diabetes mellitus.

'Cutaneous markers' of diabetes
Necrobiosis lipoidica diabeticorum
Granuloma annulare
Diabetic dermopathy ('shin spots')
Diabetic thick skin (including diabetic hand syndrome)
Acanthosis nigricans
Diabetic bullae

Complications of diabetes
Neurovascular and ischaemic skin changes and foot ulceration
Digital gangrene (due to atherosclerosis)
Disordered sweating (with autonomic neuropathy)
Increased susceptibility to skin infections:
• bacterial (boils, erythrasma)
• yeasts (candidiasis — intertrigo, perineal infections, balanitis)
• fungal dermatoses

Complications of diabetic treatment
Sulphonylureas:
• maculopapular eruptions
• Stevens–Johnson syndrome
• purpura
• photosensitivity
• erythema nodosum
• porphyria cutanea tarda
• alcohol-induced flushing with chlorpropamide ('CPAF')
Insulin:
• localized allergy (late-phase, Arthus or delayed reactions)
• systemic allergy (urticaria, anaphylaxis)
• lipoatrophy
• lipohypertrophy
• idiosyncratic reactions (pigmentation, keloid formation)

Rare associations with endocrine and other syndromes
Glucagonoma (migratory necrolytic erythema)
Cushing's syndrome (skin atrophy, striae, hirsutes)
Acromegaly (thickened skin, increased sweating)
Partial and total lipodystrophy (variable loss of subcutaneous fat)
Ataxia telangiectasia

• Diabetic thick skin includes both the rare scleroedema (affecting the neck, upper back and arms) and the common diabetic hand syndrome (cheiroarthropathy, Dupuytren's contractures, sclerosing tenosynovitis, knuckle pads and carpal tunnel syndrome). Dupuytren's contracture and Garrod's knuckle pads are shown in Figs 22.4 and 22.5. Affected patients show the 'prayer sign' (an inability to appose the palmar surfaces of the

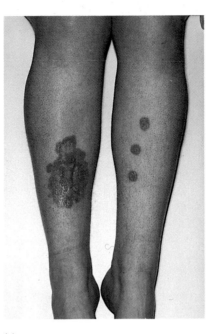

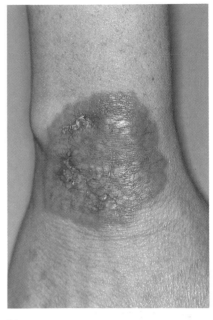

Fig. 22.1. Necrobiosis lipoidica diabeticorum. (a) A typical lesion on the front of the right shin, with three smaller areas on the left shin. (b) An area of necrobiosis with the typical yellow atrophic centre and telangiectases, on the unusual site of the dorsum of the wrist.

(a)

(b)

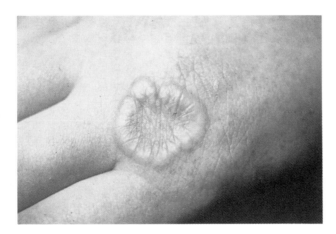

Fig. 22.2. Granuloma annulare. (Courtesy of Dr Geoffrey V. Gill.)

hand when the fingertips are pressed together).
• Acanthosis nigricans forms brown, velvety hyperkeratotic plaques in the axilla or back of the neck (Fig. 22.6). Histologically, the epidermis is extensively folded with increased melanocytes.
• There is a frequent association of acanthosis nigricans with a large heterogeneous group of disorders with the common feature of insulin resistance, ranging from asymptomatic hyperinsulinaemia to overt diabetes. Acanthosis—insulin resistance syndromes are classified into two main groups, type A (genetic defects in the insulin receptor or postreceptor mechanisms) and type B (acquired insulin resistance, due to autoantibodies

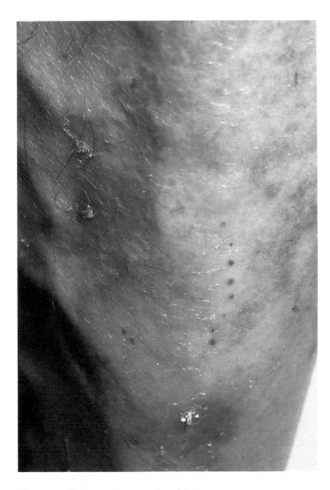

Fig. 22.3. Diabetic dermopathy ('shin spots').

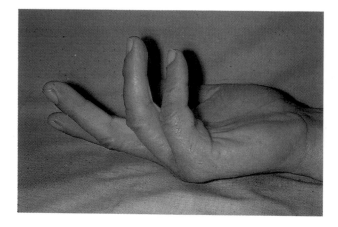

Fig. 22.4. Dupuytren's contracture in a diabetic patient with thickened skin and limited joint mobility.

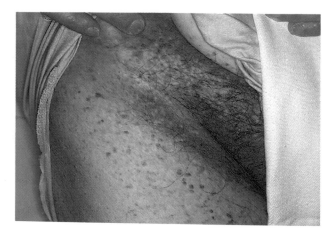

Fig. 22.6. Acanthosis nigricans in the groin.

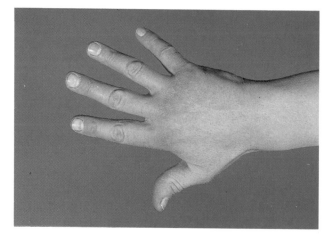

Fig. 22.5. Garrod's knuckle pads — thickening of the skin and superficial subcutaneous tissues — overlying the proximal interphalangeal joints in a patient with IDDM.

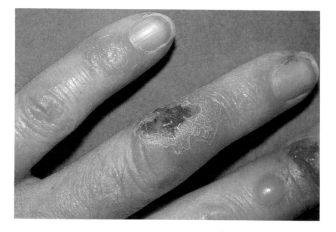

Fig. 22.7. Bullosis diabeticorum.

directed against the insulin receptor). Endocrine-associated acanthosis nigricans appears to be a true cutaneous marker, if not of overt diabetes, then at least of abnormal carbohydrate metabolism. The mechanism responsible for the development of acanthosis nigricans is uncertain, although the high circulating insulin concentrations associated with insulin resistance could promote epidermal growth.

● If necessary, the cosmetically disturbing appearance of acanthosis nigricans may be improved by applying mild peeling agents such as 5% salicylic acid in a bland cream.

● Bullosis diabeticorum usually occurs in patients with long-standing neuropathy and consists of tense blisters on a non-inflamed base which appear suddenly on the feet or hands (Fig. 22.7). The condition is very rare.

● Cutaneous complications of diabetic treatment include reactions to sulphonylurea drugs (especially first generation), insulin allergy and injection-site lipodystrophy. Figure 22.8 shows the Stevens–Johnson syndrome which may complicate the use of sulphonylureas and Fig. 22.9 illustrates lipohypertrophy due to insulin injection.

● The rare glucagonoma syndrome (associated with an A-cell pancreatic tumour) presents with a migratory erythematous eruption, with peripheral scaling and vesiculation leading to erosions and ulceration. The characteristic sites are perioral, genital and perianal.

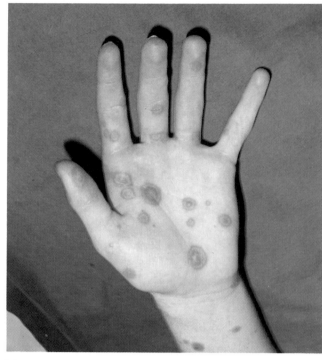

(a)

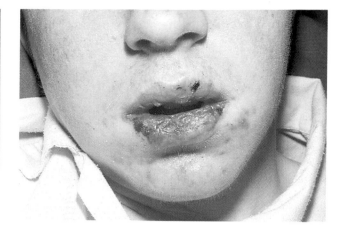

(b)

Fig. 22.8. Stevens–Johnson syndrome, showing typical 'target lesions' of erythema multiforme (a), and mouth ulceration (b). This is a rare complication of treatment with sulphonylureas.

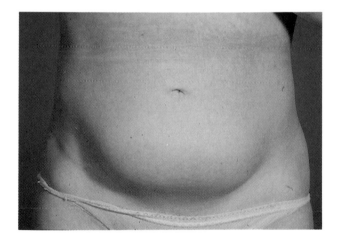

Fig. 22.9. Lipohypertrophy at site of habitual insulin injection.

23: Sexual function in diabetic men

• Impotence is the inability to achieve or sustain an erection satisfactory for sexual intercourse. It is one of the saddest complications of diabetes and is relatively common in diabetic men. However, in the UK at least, it is probably the least discussed problem related to the disease. Even though the ultimate prognosis in many cases is poor, patients will often appreciate the opportunity to discuss this once-taboo subject with their physician.

• The prevalence of impotence in diabetic men is high (up to 35%, according to one large study). Associated factors at presentation in this study were increasing age, the presence of retinopathy, and peripheral and autonomic neuropathy. There was no apparent relationship with the duration of the disease, but poor glycaemic control and excessive alcohol intake at presentation seemed to be important. In a follow-up study of the same population 5 years later, 28% of those originally potent had developed impotence and 9% of the impotent had become potent.

• It is important to differentiate 'impotence in diabetic men' from 'diabetic impotence', as the latter term implies organic disease which is essentially irreversible and untreatable. The possible causes of impotence must therefore be carefully considered in each individual case.

Physiology of normal erection and ejaculation

• The physiological complexity of the male sexual response (Fig. 23.1) underlines the many ways in which various organic and psychological factors may cause impotence.

• Erection is a parasympathetic response to psychic, visual and other stimuli acting on higher cortical centres and to reflex tactile stimulation of the genitalia. The sacral parasympathetic outflow (carried via the pudendal nerves) causes dilatation of the corporeal arteries (end-branches of the internal pudendal artery), leading to engorgement of the corpora cavernosa and corpus spongiosum. Sustained erection depends not only on increased arterial inflow but also on restriction of venous outflow from the corpora.

• Ejaculation is a sympathetic response, mediated by the presacral nerves arising from the lower part of the thoraco-lumbar sympathetic outflow, which causes contraction of the vas deferens and seminal vesicles.

• Inability to produce or sustain an erection can result from many factors which may be either related or unrelated to diabetes (Table 23.1).

Component	Interfering factors causing impotence
Psychological arousal	Depression, anxiety (including that about diabetes) Psychotropic drugs Alcohol, cannabis
Tactile input from genitalia	Peripheral neuropathy
Parasympathetic outflow	Autonomic neuropathy Various antihypertensive and other drugs
Increased arterial inflow to corpora	Atheroma of iliac or pudendal arteries
Reduced venous outflow from corpora	Venous leakage
Adequate testosterone levels	Hypogonadism

Table 23.1. Factors necessary for erection and causes of impotence.

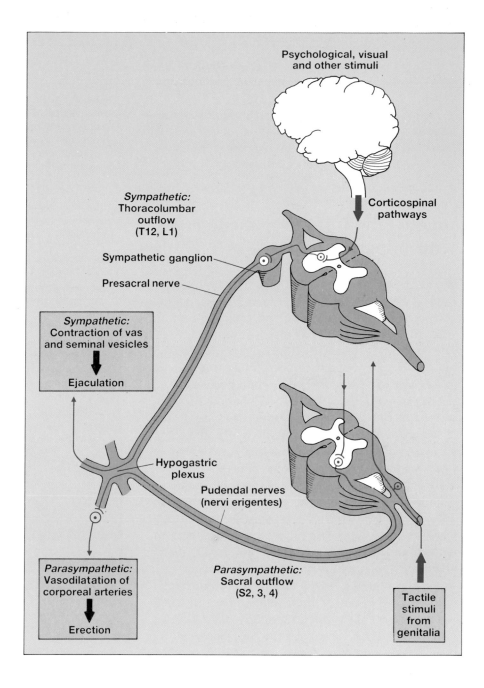

Fig. 23.1. Mechanisms regulating erection and ejaculation.

• Although a proportion of diabetic men will have irreversible organic impotence, other potentially treatable cases must be excluded. The development of impotence in any man will depend on many interrelated influences, including his marital relationship; basic personality and upbringing; cultural and personal attitudes to life and sex; tendency to anxiety or depression; presence of and response to pressure at work or at home; and the use of drugs and alcohol. The particular pathophysiological complications and psychosocial pressures of diabetes itself will be superimposed upon and will interact with this complex and delicate background.

• Psychogenic causes, often associated with anxiety and/or depression, are common; nocturnal erections are maintained and patients may respond to expert counselling.

• Autonomic neuropathy may interrupt the parasympathetic outflow which normally produces vasodilatation and engorgement of the penile corpora.

• Vascular causes of impotence include both reduced arterial inflow (through obstruction of iliac or internal pudendal arteries) and venous leakage from the corpora.

- Impotence may also be due to alcohol or cannabis abuse, to antihypertensive or psychotropic drugs, or rarely to hypogonadism.

- From the above, it is obvious that many neurological, vascular and endocrine factors may potentially be involved and may be aggravated by coexisting psychogenic problems.

Investigation of the diabetic man with impotence

- This is outlined in Table 23.2. The first step is to elicit an adequate history, concentrating on the above factors, during a free and open discussion with the patient and, ideally, with his partner. The subject is rarely mentioned spontaneously, but it is wrong for the clinician to assume that if it is not brought up, then it is not a problem. The patient should therefore be questioned directly, but it must be stressed that adequate assessment of an impotent man is a skilled task requiring special consideration and training, and is not a topic for a brief chat in a busy clinic.

- The patient will also need a full physical examination, particularly to seek evidence of autonomic and peripheral neuropathy, peripheral vascular disease (with the above reservation regarding atheroma restricted to small distal arteries), hypogonadism and alcohol abuse.

- A 'snap gauge' may demonstrate nocturnal erections which are often maintained in men whose impotence is predominantly psychogenic; however, the usefulness of this test has recently been questioned.

Management of impotence in the diabetic man

- Sympathetic counselling (ideally of both partners) is the first stage.

Table 23.2. Assessment of the diabetic man with impotence.

History and examination for evidence of
Anxiety, depression
Impact of impotence
Drug and alcohol use
Autonomic neuropathy (especially involving bladder)
Peripheral neuropathy
Peripheral vascular disease (NB: poor correlation of femoral pulses with pudendal artery patency)
Hypogonadism

Further investigations
Formal psychological assessment of patient (and partner)
Autonomic function tests
Assessment of nocturnal erections (snap-gauge)

Specialist-centre investigations
Penile blood flow
Electrophysiological tests

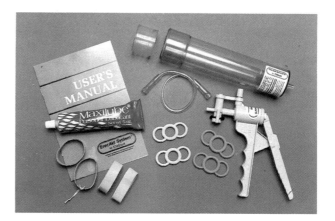

Fig. 23.2. A vacuum device to produce penile tumescence and erection.

- Treatments available for organic causes of impotence include suction devices causing passive erection (see Fig. 23.2), intracorporeal injection of vasodilators (e.g. papaverine), and surgical implantation of rigid or inflatable prostheses.

24: Spreading the load: the roles of the general practitioner and the diabetic-specialist nurse

The role of the practitioner and 'shared care'

• Diabetes is a common, chronic disease, whose optional management demands an integrated and well-coordinated effort from a number of sources. Hospital diabetic clinics clearly cannot and should not have to deal with all diabetics. General practitioners must accept the clinical challenge of the disease; indeed, many would argue that they should supervise most aspects of the diabetic patient's life, only referring to the local specialist those patients who have complications or particular problems with control.

• In Britain, the average general practice list will include about 30 diabetic patients and, because diabetes impinges on many aspects of medicine, a significant part of the general practitioner's workload can involve diabetes. General practitioners have a crucial part to play in the successful management of the condition: it is important, for instance, to know whether the woman seeking contraceptive advice, the toddler with an upper respiratory tract infection, or the older patient in heart failure has diabetes.

• 'Shared care' schemes, combining the skills of the general practitioner and the hospital physician, are an effective use of resources (Fig. 24.1).

• Most diabetic patients can be managed largely by general practitioners, although special groups (children, adolescents, pregnant women and those with specific complications or poor control) will require hospital review.

• Successful general practice management depends on a joint team approach involving the patient, his relatives, a specialist nurse, dietitian, chiropodist and the doctor, who should co-ordinate activities. There is now evidence that the diabetic patient's attitude and behaviour are crucial to good metabolic control, and education about diabetes and its treatment is a vital part of the health-care plan. Each team member must decide the various components of the education programme for which he/she is responsible, and the information given must be uniform and consistent. The practice nurse should be the patient's main contact.

• The basic requirements for setting up a diabetic clinic in a general practice are summarized in Fig. 24.2. The importance of good records and documentation cannot be over-emphasized: the cornerstone of organized diabetic care must be a register of all known diabetic patients in the practice. In the absence of a disease index, compiling such a register is a formidable task, but diabetic patients can be identified from memory, by scanning requests for repeat prescriptions, and by screening. Blood or urine glucose should be routinely checked in all newly registered patients and in those with obesity, septic lesions of any sort or leg ulceration, or a family history of diabetes.

• All patients should have a full annual review, including assessments of the cardiovascular system and feet and a fundal examination performed by an experienced person (Fig. 24.3).

• Inspection of the eyes is especially important and should be performed in hospital if the practitioner has any doubts about his/her ability to

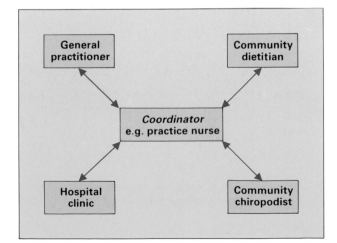

Fig. 24.1. The shared care team in general practice.

- An interested and enthusiastic general practitioner

- An easily accessible practice nurse

- A regular clinic session (protected time)

- A specialized record card

- Secretarial facilities which identify defaulters

- Close cooperation with the local hospital diabetic clinic and biochemistry laboratory

Fig. 24.2. Requirements for general practice care of diabetic patients.

identify and interpret the various stages of retinopathy. Deterioration of vision (by more than one line on the Snellen chart), or a visual acuity worse than 6/9 which is not corrected by removing refraction errors (with the patient wearing his

- Lying and standing blood pressure

- Visual acuity with refraction through a pin-hole

- Examination of fundi (dilate pupils after checking acuity)

- Foot examination

- Examination of peripheral pulses

- Screening of peripheral sensory nervous system (reflexes, light touch, pin prick); full examination if symptoms are present

- Urinalysis (a) ketones,
              (b) protein

- Blood (a) urea, creatinine, electrolytes,
         (b) fasting lipids

Fig. 24.3. A suggested annual review for general practice.

1 Simple explanation of IDDM and need for insulin

2 The patient's own insulin regimen:
  - Type(s) of insulin; mixing technique if necessary
  - Number of injections; timing relative to meals
  - Syringe: site, and special aids (pen device, 'click-count', etc.)
  - Injection technique, sites and rotation
  - Insulin storage and where to obtain supplies

3 Diabetic control:
  - Define and explain normal, too high and too low values
  - Self-monitoring using blood or urine glucose testing
  - When to test
  - Recording of results
  - What to do if values are too high or too low
  - Use of Ketostix if needed

4 The patient's own diet:
  - Choice of unrefined carbohydrate, high-fibre and low-fat foods
  - Recognition of amounts of carbohydrate
  - Regular spacing of meals
  - Ideal body weight

5 Hypoglycaemia:
  - Recognizing symptoms
  - Corrective action; need to carry sugar and identification
  - How to avoid hypoglycaemia

6 Keeping in contact:
  - Written or taped instructions
  - Contact telephone number and next planned contact

Table 24.1. 'First aid' knowledge checklist for patients with IDDM.

spectacles or looking through a pin-hole in a piece of card) should be referred for a specialist opinion.
• As mentioned above, good record keeping is essential; a 'co-operation card' or booklet provides effective communication between the practice and the hospital.
• Patient education is essential to good diabetes management; initial survival information must be followed up by a continuing educational programme.

The role of the diabetic-specialist nurse

• It is now generally accepted that diabetic people must understand their diabetes and how to manage it in order to achieve sufficiently good control to avoid the acute metabolic problems of the disease and, it is hoped, its complications. It is also now acknowledged that the diabetes specialist nurse has an essential role to play in educating, advising and counselling people with diabetes, in teaching their colleagues about the disease, and in co-ordinating the delivery of diabetes care by the hospital and/or the community.
• The Royal College of Physicians has recom-mended that, in the UK, there should be at least one diabetes specialist nurse per 100 000 population.
• In the UK, training as a diabetes specialist nurse begins with 6 months basic training in diabetes followed by a short course under the auspices of the English National Board. Various advanced courses for specialist nurses are now available.
• Home visits by the specialist nurse to supervise the initiation or stabilization of insulin treatment, or to tackle specific topics such as self-monitoring, can often avoid the need for hospital admission or out-patient attendance. Specialist nurses can therefore save considerable hospital resources and are very cost-effective.
• Perhaps the specialist nurse's most vital role is in providing and testing the patient's knowledge about diabetes. Suggested topics for IDDM and NIDDM patients are outlined in Tables 24.1–4; the gradual provision of knowledge is very crucial to prevent 'information overload' and encourage the patient's understanding and compliance.
• The nurse is also well placed to provide counselling and patients often find her more approachable than the doctor in a busy hospital clinic or general practice.

Table 24.2. More advanced knowledge check-list for patients with IDDM.

1 Insulin regimen:
  • Action profile and time-course of patient's insulin(s)
  • Reasons why blood glucose levels rise or fall
  • How and when to alter the dose

2 Intercurrent events:
  • Exercise, parties
  • Minor illness; major illness with fever, anorexia, vomiting
  • How to recognize ketoacidosis
  • Warning signs to call for help

3 Chronic complications of diabetes:
  • Long-term complications
  • Positive action to try to avoid these
  • Specific complications and their treatment, e.g. foot care
  • Need for annual review and what to expect

4 Miscellaneous:
  • Driving
  • Insurance
  • Employment
  • Smoking and alcohol
  • Holidays and travel
  • Genetic counselling, contraception, pregnancy
  • Membership of British Diabetic Association or other national associations and patient groups
  • New advances in diabetes care or research

Table 24.3. 'First aid' check-list for patients with NIDDM.

1 Simple explanation of NIDDM

2 The patient's own diet:
   - Choice of unrefined carbohydrate, high-fibre and low-fat foods
   - Recognition of amounts of carbohydrate
   - Regular spacing of meals
   - Ideal body weight and targets for weight loss

3 The patient's own drug treatment
   - Mode of action
   - Possible side-effects
   - Dosage and schedule

4 Diabetic control ⎫
5 Hypoglycaemia ⎬ as for IDDM (Table 24.1).
6 Keeping contact ⎭

Table 24.4. More advanced knowledge check-list for patients with NIDDM.

1 Treatment regimen:
   - Reasons why blood glucose levels fall or rise
   - How to recognize need for a change in dosage

2 Intercurrent events ⎫
3 Chronic complications of diabetes ⎬ as for IDDM (Table 24.2)
4 Miscellaneous ⎭

Index

Abbreviations used in the index: DM, diabetes mellitus; IDDM, insulin-dependent diabetes mellitus; NIDDM, non-insulin-dependent diabetes mellitus.